SICKLE STATES: CLINICAL FEATURES IN WEST AFRICANS

This book is dedicated to E.N.B.

SICKLE STATES:
CLINICAL FEATURES
IN WEST AFRICANS

ROGER A. LEWIS M.D.
Professor of Pharmacology Ghana Medical School, Accra

GHANA UNIVERSITIES PRESS
ACCRA
1970

Ghana Universities Press
P.O. Box 4219
Accra, Ghana

PRINTED AND BOUND IN ENGLAND BY
HAZELL WATSON AND VINEY LTD
AYLESBURY, BUCKS

Contents

Contents

List of Figures

List of Tables

I : Introduction

THOUSANDS of years ago, in the tropical part of Africa, malaria was rampant. A large proportion of infants died of this disease before they had a chance to develop sufficient immunity to keep the infection under control. As a result, malaria has left its mark on the African red cell (92).

The malaria parasite attacks the red cells of the blood, in fact, lives and reproduces inside these cells. The chief constituent of the red cells is the pigment hemoglobin, a protein composed of four units, each containing an atom of iron, a porphyrin complex, and a polypeptide chain of more than 100 amino acids (81).

A mutation or change in the genetic pattern controlling the formation of hemoglobin must have taken place. The change led to the substitution of a different amino acid in one of the 100 places in one pair of the polypeptide chains of the hemoglobin molecule (64).

As a result of this simple change in the chemical structure of hemoglobin, the disc shaped red cell is liable to undergo an alteration in shape. As the oxygen level of the blood falls, the discs take on the shape of an oat grain, a holly leaf, or a farmer's sickle (41).

The inheritance of S hemoglobin follows the laws of Mendel. Each person inherits two genes for the character, one from the mother and one from the father. With most inherited characteristics, if unlike genes are inherited, one of them will predominate and determine the characteristic. In the case of sickle hemoglobin, the single gene is not dominant or recessive. The individual inheriting normal adult hemoglobin A from one parent and S hemoglobin from the other parent, will manufacture red cells containing almost half sickle and half normal hemoglobins. This individual is said to be heterozygous in inheritance (genotype) and in body composition (phenotype) (64).

Almost one fourth of the people living in tropical Africa have sickle cell trait (126). It is obvious that this characteristic must have had value to the individual posessing it, or the genetic change would have remained rare.

It has been shown that the young child with sickle cell trait has partial protection against malaria (1). The number of parasites in the blood remains at a lower level than in the young child with normal hemoglobin. The young child with sickle cell trait is less likely to develop a paucity of red cells as a result of frequent attacks of malaria and enlargement of the spleen from the same cause (101). The child with sickle cell trait is less likely to develop an attack of malaria affecting the brain, which is often fatal (121).

Thus, at times and in places where malaria is rampant, children with a normal hemoglobin pattern will have a higher mortality while a greater proportion of those with sickle cell trait will survive. This increases the proportion of individuals in the community with sickle cell trait and explains the high incidence of this peculiarity of the African red cell (92).

Unfortunately, wherever sickle cell trait is common, there will be some individuals born with two genes for S hemoglobin. These children are unable to form any normal hemoglobin and can make only S and F hemoglobins. The genotype is SS and the phenotype S with a small amount of F. Such individuals have sickle cell anemia, the most severe type of sickle cell disease.

Persons with sickle cell anemia, as the name implies, are anemic. They are prone to infections and suffer from rheumatic pains. Such infants fail to thrive and many die before reaching the tender age of two years.

The disadvantage to society of having some individuals with sickle cell anemia is the price paid by the population for the advantage gained by having a large number of individuals with sickle cell trait. Fortunately, the number of persons with sickle cell anemia is much smaller than the number with sickle cell trait. Furthermore, with the improvement of medical facilities and the rise in standard of living in Africa, children with sickle cell disease are now having a longer and more comfortable life (84).

In Ghana and Upper Volta there are also many individuals with hemoglobin C trait (1). In Southeast Asia there are many persons with hemoglobin E trait (126). And, along the shore of the Mediterranean there are many individuals who have inherited thalassemia trait, a peculiarity of hemoglobin formation that leads to the formation of smaller than normal red cells and increased amounts of hemoglobins A_2 and F (168).

There is an unrelated abnormality which affects African red cells. This has nothing to do with hemoglobin although it is an abnormality of the red cell. The red cells are living bodies that gain their energy from the sugar glucose. In the red cell the glucose is usually attached to another substance, phosphate ion. Glucose contains 6 carbons and the phosphate ion is attached to the last carbon giving rise to the designation glucose-6-phosphate. Most of the glucose-6-phosphate or G-6-P is split up and reformed without loss of glucose or consumption of oxygen, the anaerobic pathway. But a small proportion of the G-6-P is oxidized and destroyed with consumption of oxygen, the aerobic pathway. For this pathway, an adequate supply of catalytic agent or enzyme called glucose-6-phosphate dehydrogenase (G-6-P D) is required (15).

The enzyme G-6-P D is deficient although not entirely absent from the red cells of almost one fifth of the population of tropical Africa (127). A similar, but more severe deficiency affects the red cells of people living in other tropical areas. In fact, it has been estimated that there are over 100 million people in the world with a deficiency of this enzyme (53). Since deficiency of the enzyme occurs in the same areas as abnormal hemoglobins and thalassemia, it is assumed that the enzyme defect may also play a role in protection against malaria. However, since the disadvantages associated with enzyme lack are small compared with the drawbacks of sickle cell anemia, the advantage in malaria protection may also be very small (92).

The inheritance of G-6-P D defect is sex linked so that males inherit this peculiarity from their mothers, while females may inherit it from either or both parents. In males the enzyme is present in normal amounts or is grossly deficient. In females an intermediate stage is more common.

Infants inheriting the enzyme defect may become jaundiced shortly after birth. If the jaundice increases there may be brain damage and death. Persons with the defect have a greater tendency to become jaundiced when the liver is damaged as in viral hepatitis (29). The ingestion of certain drugs such as primaquine may also cause a severe hemolytic anemia in such individuals (76). In fact, deficiency of the enzyme G-6-P D is sometimes referred to as primaquine type sensitivity. In the Mediterranean type of G-6-P D deficiency the ingestion of fava beans produces the same type of hemolytic reaction which is known as favism (15).

Unless and until the presence of normal enzyme activity has become established, full doses of the antimalarial, primaquine, should not be given to Africans or persons of African descent (76).

Two derangements of the red cell have been mentioned, abnormal hemoglobins and G-6-P D defect. Both of these abnormalities carry with them potential disadvantages. There is another peculiarity of the

African red cell which has an advantage. This consists of a high incidence of an immune type of reaction which is detected by mixing red
cells with serum obtained from a rhesus type monkey. In Europe and
North America, there are many women with a negative rhesus reaction.
and if the unborn child has a positive rhesus reaction there is a danger
to the pregnancy (171). Most African women as well as men and their
children show a rhesus positive reaction (103). In fact, rhesus negative
individuals are one third as common in Africans as in Europeans. As a
result, there are very few instances of a pregnancy being interrupted or
ending with the death of the child due to rhesus incompatibility (45).

There are two other peculiarities of the African red cell which
remain unexplained. One is the marked prevalence of target cells, red
cells with the hemoglobin concentrated at the periphery, which can be
explained in some cases by iron deficiency and in some by the presence
of abnormal hemoglobins (34). The other peculiarity is the resistance
of African red cells to infection with *Plasmodium vivax* malaria.

Some knowledge of the peculiarities of the African red cells is
useful, not only to doctors and nurses, but also to authorities dealing
with medical education and research, public health and marriage
counseling.

II : Hemoglobin

THE HEMOGLOBIN of the red cell performs vital functions, carrying oxygen from the lungs to the tissues and facilitating the transport of carbon dioxide from the tissues to the lungs. The red cells are one thousand times more numerous than the white cells and constitute half of the volume of the circulating blood (171).

One third of the weight of the red cell is due to its hemoglobin content, the other two thirds being chiefly water. It is remarkable that so much hemoglobin can be held in solution. In fact, when the hemoglobin is abnormal there is a tendency for it to come out of solution (53).

When blood is fully oxygenated it has a bright red colour and when oxygen is lost or the hemoglobin is reduced it has a bluish colour. When oxygenated hemoglobin is further oxidized, methemoglobin is formed and this has a chocolate brown colour. All of the abnormal hemoglobins except methemoglobin are subject to reversible oxygenation.

The normal and abnormal hemoglobins have the same iron atoms and the same porphyrin complexes. They differ only in the amino acid chains, see Figure I. Every normal hemoglobin has two pairs of identical chains. In adult or A hemoglobin there are two alpha and two beta chains. Normal adults have up to 3 per cent of A_2 hemoglobin which has two alpha and two delta chains. In the condition known as beta thalassemia there is a scarcity of beta chains so that there is an excess of A_2 (81).

The blood of the unborn child contains chiefly fetal or F hemoglobin. During the first year of life this is gradually replaced by adult or A hemoglobin (161). But F hemoglobin may reappear in certain blood disorders such as sickle cell anemia ,beta thalassemia, persistent fetal hemoglobin gene (94), leukemia, and the rare genetic abnormality, trisomy D (119). Fetal hemoglobin has two alpha and two gamma chains. The absence of beta chains makes it an easily synthesized hemoglobin in beta thalassemia. However, in alpha thalassemia there is a scarcity of alpha chains and instead of F hemoglobin there may be either or both H and Barts hemoglobin which do not contain alpha chains (81).

Summarizing at this point, each normal person is capable of

normal hemoglobins

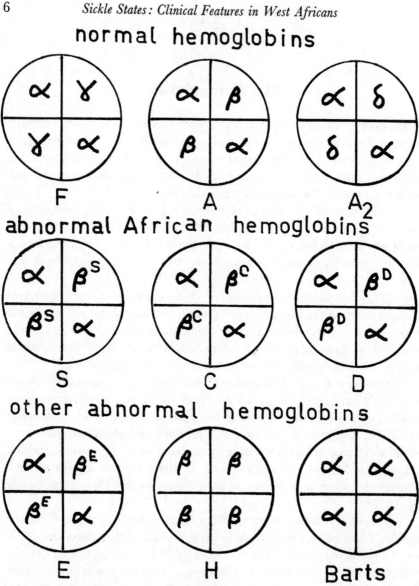

FIGURE I

making alpha, beta, gamma and delta chains. In early life alpha$_2$-gamma$_2$ or F hemoglobin predominates. In later life there is 97 per cent of A hemoglobin which is alpha$_2$beta$_2$. Adults also have about $2\frac{1}{2}$ per cent of A$_2$ or alpha$_2$delta$_2$ hemoglobin as well as $\frac{1}{2}$ per cent of F hemoglobin. In beta thalassemia there is difficulty in forming beta chains so that there is a rise of A$_2$ and F hemoglobins (168).

Most of the abnormal hemoglobins that are widely prevalent result from a mutation of the beta chain (81). Usually only one amino acid is exchanged, see Table I. There are two cases on record, hemo-

TABLE I

BETA CHAIN (POLYPEPTIDE) CHANGES IN HEMOGLOBIN VARIANTS

Area where found	Name of hemoglobin	Place of change	Amino acid lost	Amino acid gained	Change in charge
W. Africa	C	6	Glutamic	Lysine	+ +
S.E. Asia	E	26	Glutamic	Lysine	+ +
Africa	S	6	Glutamic	Valine	+
W. Africa	G$_{accra}$	79	Aspartic	Asparagine	+
W. Africa	D$_{ibadan}$	87	Threonine	Lysine	+
India	D$_{punjab}$	121	Glutamic	Glycine	+
Africa	J$_{baltimore}$	16	Glycine	Aspartic	−
Africa	N$_{baltimore}$	95	Lysine	Glutamic	− −

globin Freiberg and hemoglobin Leiden in which an amino acid was merely dropped out, and this must have happened frequently during the course of evolution of the various polypeptide chains whose similarity suggests a common origin (63).

From Table I it may be seen that the exchange of an amino acid can lead to the loss or gain of one or two electrons. Since it is the electric charge on the hemoglobin molecule that determines its rate of migration under the influence of an electric current (electrophoresis), it would be difficult to detect a hemoglobin with a change in amino acid if there were no change in the electric charge.

Loss of electrons makes the rate of migration at alkaline pH slower. Under these conditions hemoglobins C and E are among the slowest moving hemoglobins, see Figure II. Hemoglobin S moves more slowly than A but more rapidly than C. It is important to note that hemoglobins S and D have undergone the same change in electric charge which explains the fact that at alkaline pH they have the same electrophoretic mobility. On the other hand, hemoglobins J, N, I and H with an increase in electrons move more rapidly than hemoglobin A (81).

The easiest, cheapest and most rapid method of electrophoresis employs a strip of paper or cellulose acetate, see Figure III. On this strip it is possible to see the normal electrophoretic pattern AA, the pattern of sickle cell trait AS, and the pattern of sickle cell anemia SS. A trace of F hemoglobin can be seen below the SS band in sickle cell anemia (81).

+ ←————— origin -

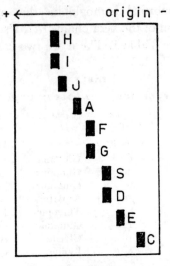

FIGURE II

Schematic representation of relative mobility of individual hemoglobins at pH 8·6.
(From Smith, C. H.: The Abnormal Hemoglobins: Clinical and Hematologic
Aspects, *J. Pediat.* **50**:91, 1957.)

In order to identify the polypetide alterations in the hemoglobin
mutants, a separation of peptides and amino acids must be made after
breaking up the chain. This is accomplished by means of a technique
which goes under the name popularized by criminal investigation
agencies, finger printing. This is a two dimensional chart made by
electrophoretic separation on one axis and chromatographic separation
at right angles (63).

The finger print of hemoglobin A is given in Figure IV and that
of S in Figure V. It may be seen that there is one spot characteristic of
A that is lacking in S and that something new has been added in S.
This change has been identified as the loss of glutamic acid and its
replacement by valine (38).

Summarizing the situation with respect to the common abnormal
hemoglobins, these have arisen by the replacement of one amino acid
in a pair of polypeptide chains, usually the beta chains. This exchange
of amino acids leads to a change in the electric charge of the hemoglobin molecule and permits separation and identification by electrophoresis. For a complete analysis of structure of a new hemoglobin it is
necessary to hydrolyze the polypeptide chain and to identify the various
fragments by a two dimensional map or finger print.

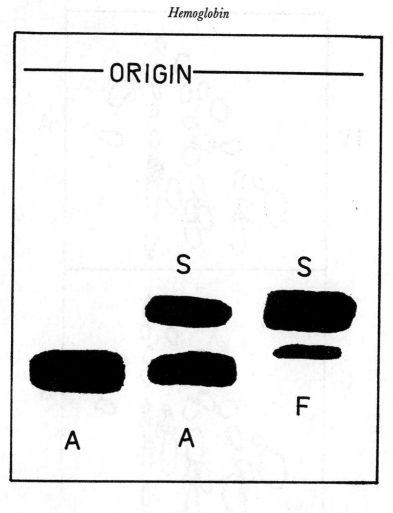

FIGURE III

Paper electrophoresis of (1) normal hemoglobin, (2) sickle-cell trait, (3) sickle-cell anemia (barbiturate buffer pH 8·9). *Note:* The hemoglobin S in the sickle cell trait is only about 40 per cent of the total. The patient with sickle cell anemia possesses some hemoglobin F but no hemoglobin A.

The chief function of hemoglobin is the transport of oxygen. The sigmoid form of the oxygen dissociation curve of hemoglobin permits it to be completely oxygenated in the lungs and to give off most of the oxygen at the oxygen tension existing in the tissues. The shape of this curve results from the presence of 4 rather than 1 oxygen atom in the

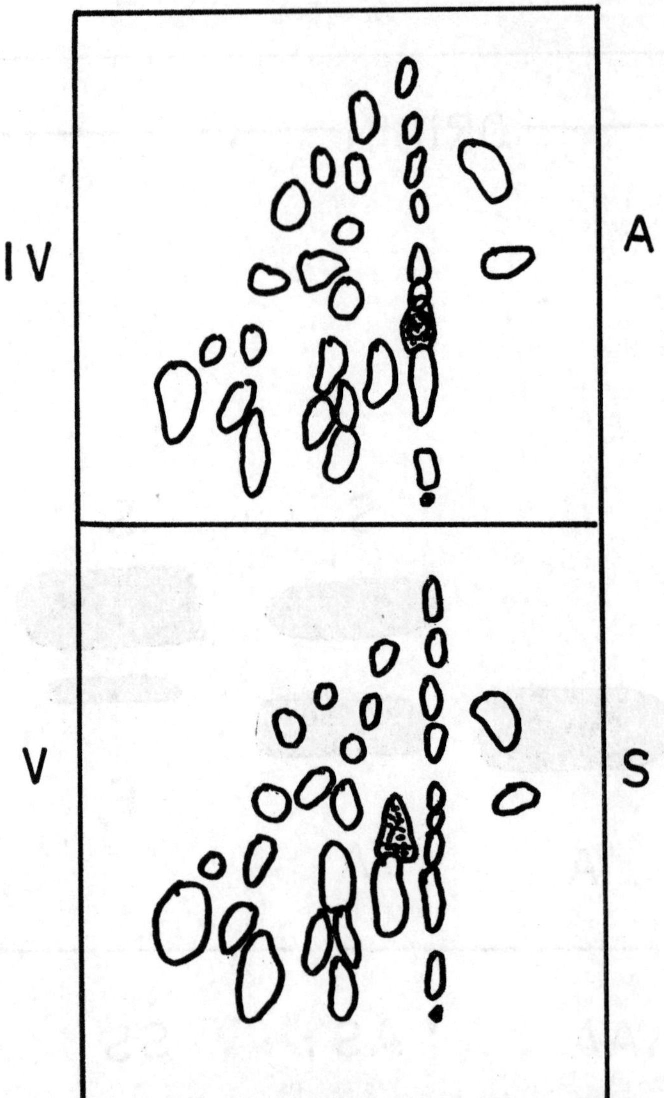

FIGURE IV

"Fingerprint pattern" of normal hemoglobin. Outline tracings of polypeptide fragments derived from hemoglobin by tryptic digestion. Spatial dispersion of the polypeptide fragments is result of subjecting the digest to electrophoresis followed by cross dimension chromatography. (From Ingram, V. M., *Nature* **178**:792, 1956)

FIGURE V

"Fingerprint pattern" of sickle hemoglobin. Position of abnormal polypeptide fragment (the sickle peptide, now designated β, see Table 1) is indicated by cross-hatched area. Its displacement relative to position of comparable peptide of the normal indicates dissimilarity in charge and composition. (From Ingram, V. M., *Nature* **178**:792, 1956) molecule. The oxygen atoms are given off, one by one, the removal of one facilitating the removal of the next (117).

It is important to know if a chemical change in the structure of hemoglobin affects the oxygen dissociation curve. Recent experiments using whole blood or red cells rather than dilute solutions of hemoglobin have shown that the oxygen dissociation curve is changed (12). In the case of S hemoglobin the curve is shifted to the left as if the solution were more alkaline, see Figure VI. This enables the tissues to obtain

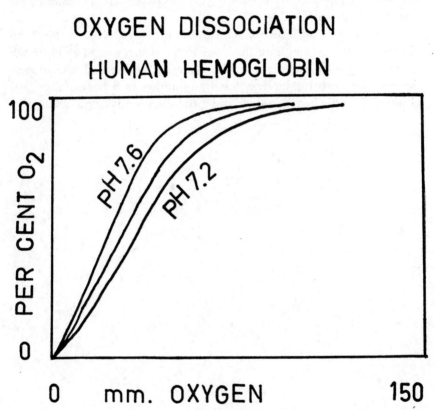

FIGURE VI

Oxygen dissociation curves of human hemoglobin at various pH values

more oxygen. As a result the patient with sickle cell anemia and a low hemoglobin level is able to deliver as much oxygen to the tissues as a normal individual. The reverse holds true in some of the rare hemoglobinopathies where polycythemia develops.

Returning to Figure VI, it may be seen that the oxygen dissociation curve fluctuates with the hydrogen ion concentration or its negative logarithm, the pH. In the tissues where carbon dioxide is produced, the hydrogen ion concentration rises and the pH falls leading to the release of more oxygen. In the lungs the carbon dioxide is removed and this gives the hemoglobin a greater affinity for oxygen (53). In the tissues where oxygen is given off, the spatial configuration of the polypeptide chains is altered and the hemoglobin is capable of binding or neutralizing more carbon dioxide. Just as removal of carbon dioxide gives hemoglobin a greater affinity for oxygen, so oxygenation facilitates the removal of carbon dioxide.

The complex structure of hemoglobin is thus reflected in its special ability to carry oxygen from the lungs to the tissues and to enhance the carriage of carbon dioxide from the tissues to the lungs. These properties are enhanced rather than lost by mutation to S hemoglobin (12) although in some hemoglobinopathies the situation is aggravated.

III : Anemia

BY DEFINITION, anemia means a lower than normal level of hemoglobin in the blood. This level can be measured colorimetrically after dissolution or hemolysis of the red cells. The hemoglobin level should be expressed in grams per 100 ml. of blood rather than as the percentage of a mythical normal value (171).

The hemoglobin level is reflected by the number of red cells, although a marked change in the average size of the red cells can make for a significant discrepancy between the red cell count and the hemoglobin level. In addition the red cell count is less accurate than the hemoglobin level measured colorimetrically. The count is expressed in millions per cubic millimeter.

The hemoglobin level is also reflected in the volume of packed red cells or hematocrit which is estimated by centrifugation of the blood. Here again, but to a lesser extent, a marked change in the average size of the red cells, or a low hemoglobin concentration in the red cells, can make for a significant discrepancy between the value of the hemoglobin level and the hematocrit. The latter is expressed in ml. per 100 ml. blood or per cent.

Because of the variations between the hemoglobin level, red cell count and hematocrit, the terms MCV or mean corpuscular volume, MCH or mean corpuscular hemoglobin and MCHC or mean corpuscular hemoglobin concentration have been introduced (171). These indices are defined as follows:

MCV = 10 (hematocrit in per cent/red cells in millions)
MCH = 10 (hemoglobin gm. per 100 ml./red cells millions)
MCHC = 100 (hemoglobin gm. per 100 ml./hematocrit in per cent).

For practical purposes the degree of anemia can be expressed by giving the hemoglobin level, the hematocrit or the red cell count. Microscopic examination of the blood film will usually reveal the presence or absence of abnormally large or abnormally small red cells, as well as less than normal hemoglobin content when this occurs (171).

Returning to a consideration of the hemoglobin level, it is important to note that at birth the figure is very high, 20 gm. per 100 ml. During the first two years of life the level gradually falls to 11. After that there is then a gradual rise to the normal adult value of 14 for women and

16 for men (148). However, during pregnancy there may be a fall of 1–2 gm. per 100 ml. in the hemoglobin level. Thus, the degree of anemia must be compared with the normal level in relation to age and sex, see Figure VII (171). In sickle cell anemia the hemoglobin level in the steady state rarely exceeds 10 although in sickle cell hemoglobin C disease the hemoglobin level may reach the normal value (53).

Once the presence of anemia has been established, it is important

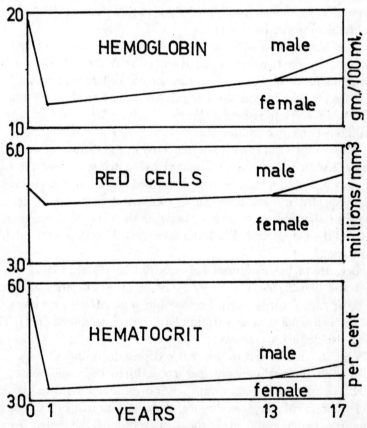

FIGURE VII

Normal curve for hemoglobin, red cells and volumes of packed red cells, from birth to old age. The mean values are heavily outlined. The range of variation is indicated by dotted lines for hemoglobin, interrupted lines for red cell count and dotted interrupted lines for volume of packed red cells. The scales for hemoglobin, red cell count and volume of packed red cells are similar and therefore the relative changes in these three values are apparent on inspection. The scale for age, however, is progressively altered. (Derived from the data of Williamson, Appleton, Haden and Neff, Merritt and Davidson, Poncher, Guest, Osgood and Baker, Kato, Mugrage and Andresen and Wintrobe.)

to know if the red cells are larger than normal in size (macrocytic), normal in size (normocytic), or smaller than normal in size (microcytic). If the cells are small in size and also have a lower than normal hemoglobin concentration the anemia is microcytic and hypochromic (171).

Microscopic examination of the ordinary stained smear of the blood not only reveals abnormalities in the size of the red cells, the presence or absence of nucleated red cells, but also variations in the shape of the red cells. Some of the changes in shape which may be seen are illustrated in Figure VIII. The presence of crenated cells or rouleaux is not abnormal. The Figure does not illustrate target cells which are so designated because of the concentration of hemoglobin at the periphery of the cell. Such red cells are frequent when there is iron deficiency or when there is an abnormal type of hemoglobin, especially hemoglobin C (34). Furthermore, the holly leaf and sickle shaped cells which are illustrated are characteristic of blood which has been allowed to stand, although oat shaped cells may be found in the fresh smear (59).

The majority of macrocytic anemias in the tropics are due to lack of folic acid or vitamin B_{12} in the diet or difficulty in the absorption of these vitamins (36). At certain seasons and in certain parts of Africa the deficiency is especially likely to occur in children, pregnant women and patients with sickle cell anemia (167). Table II correlates the type of anemia with the probable causes.

Chronic malarial infection often leads to anemia of the normocytic type. Bacterial infections may also cause normocytic anemia while other chronic diseases usually result in a microcytic type of anemia. Iron deficiency is characterized by a hypochromic microcytic picture (173).

Most of the anemias caused by abnormal hemoglobin diseases are of the normocytic type. In thalassemia and sickle cell thalassemia there may be a microcytic anemia (168). However, the characteristic feature of the anemias due to abnormal hemoglobins is the increased rate of production and destruction of red cells and a shortening of the life span of the red cells. This causes an increase in the percentage of immature forms, nucleated red cells and reticulocytes, and an increase in the by-products of hemoglobin destruction, especially bilirubin, which is responsible for the yellow discolouration of the eyes, serum and urine (156).

Deficiency of the enzyme G-6-P D may, under certain conditions, lead to a normocytic anemia. During acute phases there is increased

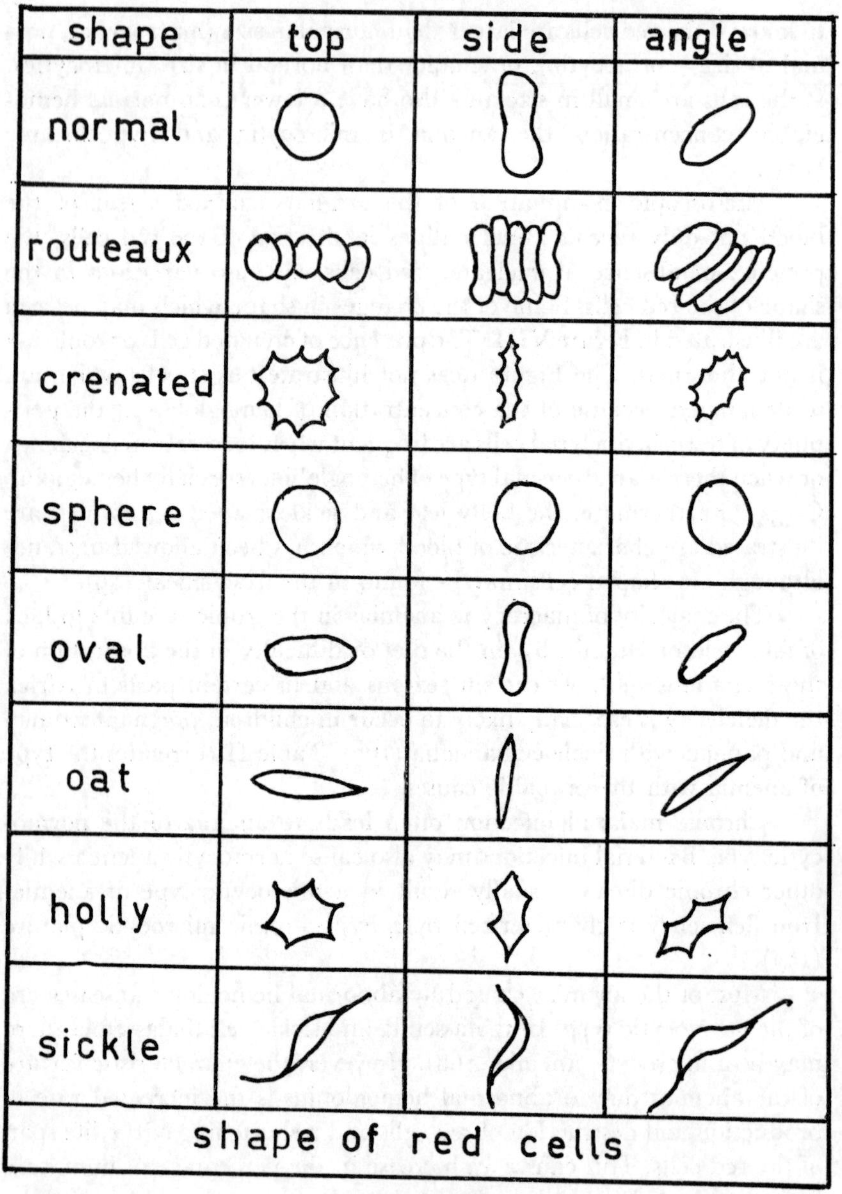

shape	top	side	angle
normal			
rouleaux			
crenated			
sphere			
oval			
oat			
holly			
sickle			

shape of red cells

FIGURE VIII

destruction of red cells and subsequently increased production, see Figure IX (3).

The symptoms of anemia are weakness, fatigue, and shortness of breath on exertion. The signs are pallor of the mucous membranes and

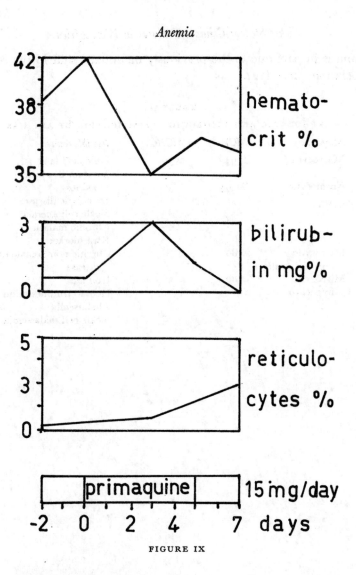

FIGURE IX

nail beds, the presence of cardiac murmurs, and if the anemia is severe the heart rate is elevated. Severe anemia lowers the body resistance to infections and may eventually lead to cardiac enlargement and then cardiac failure. Patients who have had anemia for a long time seem to get accustomed to a lower than normal level of hemoglobin so that a sudden fall to a similar level in a normal person causes more severe symptoms. For example, the patient with sickle cell anemia may look and feel quite well with a hemoglobin level half that of normal. This facility of getting along with a low hemoglobin level in sickle cell anemia is in part due to the previously mentioned shift in the oxygen dissociation curve (12).

TABLE II

MORPHOLOGIC AND ETIOLOGIC CLASSIFICATION OF ANEMIAS

Morphology	MCV	MCHC	Possible causes
Macrocytic	>94	>30	Folic acid lack
			Vitamin B_{12} lack
Normocytic	80–94	>30	Blood loss
			Hemolytic diseases
			Sickle cell anemia
			Chronic malaria
			Kwashiorkor
Microcytic normochromic	<80	>30	Chronic non-hematologic disease
Microcytic hypochromic	<80	<30	Iron lack
			Hookworm infestation
			Thalassemia
			Sickle cell thalassemia

IV : Malaria

SINCE young children with sickle cell trait are less susceptible to malaria than normal children of the same age (1) one might reasonably expect that children with sickle cell anemia and other types of sickle cell disease would also enjoy some protection against malaria. Paradoxically, these individuals suffer more from malaria than normal children. This paradox stems from the fact that almost any type of infection, however slight, upsets the balance in the patient with sickle cell disease and may lead to a crisis or worsening of the condition (37). In West Africa, malaria frequently occurs in children with sickle cell anemia (58) and is one of the most common causes of crisis. A typical instance of this phenomenon is shown in Figure X which illustrates the temperature chart of a young adult with sickle cell thalassemia who was admitted to the hospital with a hemolytic crisis that continued until it was discovered that her blood contained parasites of P. falciparum and chloroquine was administered.

There are four species of Plasmodium that affect the human, see Table III. Of these, P. falciparum is the most prevalent in Africa and

TABLE III

TYPES OF PLASMODIUM AND RESULTANT MALARIA INFECTION

Plasmodium	Infection	Prevalence in Africa	Exoeryth. cycle	Cerebral* malaria
Falciparum	Malignant tertian	++++	o	+
Vivax	Benign tertian	+	+	o
Ovale	Ovale tertian	++	+	o
Malariae	Quartan	++	+	o

* Also applies to blackwater fever.

the species most likely to cause anemia or to trigger off a crisis in sickle cell disease. It is the only species of the parasite that can cause cerebral malaria and blackwater fever (136). Fortunately, P. falciparum does not have a secondary exoerythrocytic cycle in the liver, so that when a primary attack is successfully treated there is no possibility of relapse.

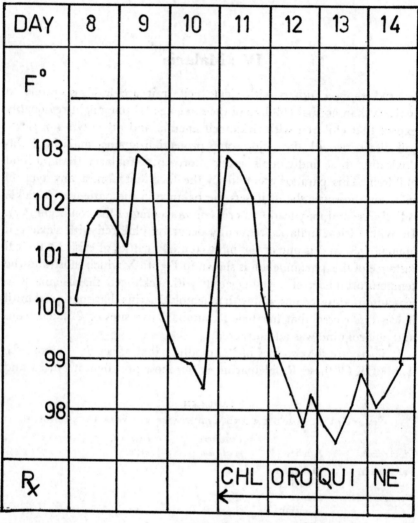

FIGURE X

Of course, a recrudescence may follow inadequate treatment or treatment of a resistant strain and there is always the possibility of reinfection (125). The other species of Plasmodium have a secondary exoerythrocytic cycle so that relapse is likely to occur unless treatment is supplemented by the administration of primaquine (172).

The species of malaria parasite can be determined by examination of the blood smear containing trophozoites or gametocytes. P. falciparum produces many more merozoites from a single schizont than other species of malarial parasite, accounting for the heavier and more severe infection. It may be noted that a single negative blood examination for parasites, does not exclude the diagnosis of malaria in view of the periodicity of the infection. Furthermore, the finding of parasites in the blood does not always signify a clinical attack as the immune individual is often a symptomless carrier (136).

The clinical diagnosis of malaria is important as it may be necessary to initiate therapy before a laboratory report can be obtained. The most important sign of malaria is the fever which may show a peak at one, two or three day intervals according to the species of parasite. But the most characteristic finding is fever out of all proportion to other symptoms which may be only lassitude, headache, anorexia and malaise. Enlargement and tenderness of the spleen are characteristic, but may be absent. Anemia, a reduced leukocyte count and pigment in the leukocytes suggests a long standing infection. A prompt response to antimalaria treatment, as illustrated in Figure X, is confirmatory evidence of malaria infection.

The clinical picture of malaria depends in part on the degree of immunity which, although it is not absolute, can often lead to clinical control in the absence of specific treatment. This immunity is reflected in the high level of globulin in the plasma of adults living in the tropics. The immunity is present at birth and declines during the first two years of life, and also during pregnancy. This accounts for the high incidence of malaria in children and pregnant women. Thus, the partial protection against malaria that is associated with sickle cell trait is best seen in children under the age of five years (92).

Cerebral malaria is a form of severe malignant tertian disease. It starts with fever, severe headache, and drowsiness followed by psychological and neurological disturbances including meningismus, convulsions and paralysis, ending with coma. The parasitemia is very heavy and there may be anemia. Cerebral malaria may end fatally in the absence of energetic treatment which includes the parenteral administration of antimalarials (172).

Blackwater fever is a complication of malignant tertian infection that is characterized by the appearance of hemoglobin, red cells and derived pigments in the urine which takes on a very dark colour. Although this reaction may occur prior to the administration of antimalarial drugs it has been seen more frequently after the use of quinine. The presence of G-6-P D deficiency would be expected to predispose to such a reaction but the incidence of this complication is quite rare, compared with the frequency of malaria in individuals with the enzyme defect.

Repeated attacks of malaria can lead to anemia and enlargement of the spleen with retardation in growth and development. The picture may be complicated by malnutrition or other infections. Nevertheless, the spleen rate can be used as an index of the prevalence of malaria if it is estimated in children 2 to 9 years of age and weighted by multiplying the number of individuals in each spleen class by the class number as defined in Figure XI (125). Other indices of the prevalence

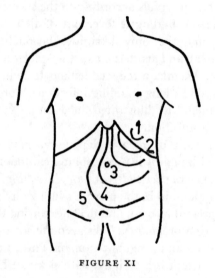

FIGURE XI

of malaria are furnished from hospital or clinic statistics of morbidity and mortality, or by estimating the number of children between the age of 2 and 9 who have positive smears for malaria (125). The degree of anemia cannot be taken as an index of malaria infection since many other factors may be involved, but when antimalaria drugs are given to children over a period of several months, there is a rise in the hemoglobin level.

In view of the high prevalence of malaria and the difficulties which have been encountered in controlling the anopheline mosquito responsible for its transmission there is a need for drugs to treat and prevent the disease, especially in individuals with sickle cell disease (58). There is a wide choice of drugs which affect different stages of the life cycle of the parasite, and effectiveness varies with the species of parasite and degree of drug resistance that has developed in the strain,

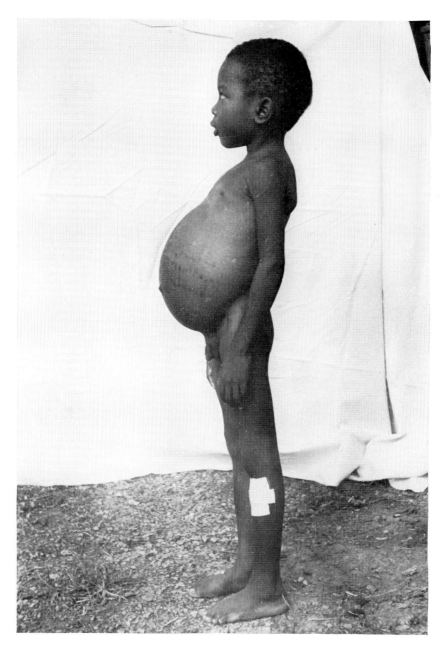

FIGURE XV

Hypersplenism in Sickle Cell Thalassemia

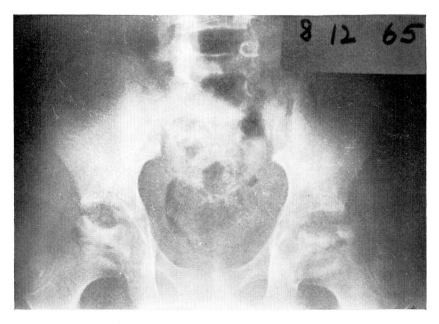

FIGURE XXXIV

Bilateral aseptic necrosis of head of femur in a child eight years old

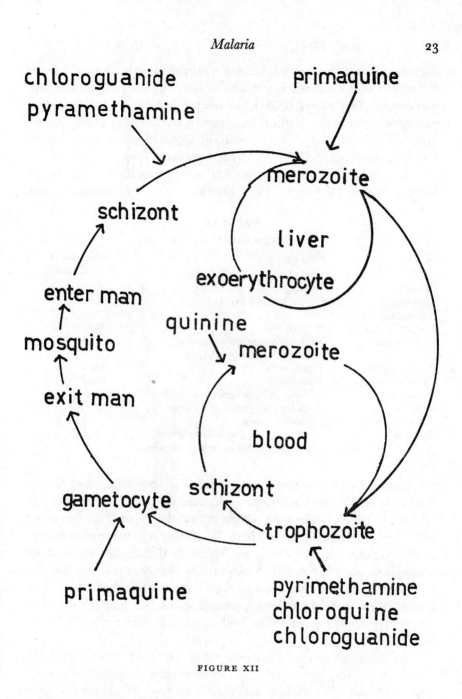

FIGURE XII

see Figure XII (83). Pyrimethamine and chloroguanide act too slowly to be used in treatment but are effective in the prophylaxis of non-resistant strains. Primaquine is the only drug which is gametocidal in falciparum infections but this form of treatment is only directed against the spread of the disease. Regardless of the drug used for clinical suppression, vivax malaria is likely to relapse because of the secondary exoerythrocytic cycle. Radical cure can be obtained by giving primaquine along with drugs used for clinical suppression but then there is a risk of hemolysis in G-6-P D deficient patients (76).

The drugs used for the treatment and prevention of malaria are listed in Table IV (100) (172). Quinine, which lost popularity with

TABLE IV

ANTI-MALARIA DRUGS

Name	*Chief uses*	*Hemolysis in G-6-P D defect*
Quinine	Treatment of resistant cases	Slight if any
Chloroquine Amodiaquine	Treatment and prophylaxis	None
Pyrimethamine	Prophylaxis	None
Trimethoprim	With sulfone or sulfonamides in treatment and prophylaxis	None
Chloroguanide	Prophylaxis	None
Chlorproguanil	Prophylaxis	None
Primaquine	Radical cure and epidemic control	Severe
Sulfalene Sulfisoxazole	With trimethoprim for treatment of resistant cases	Slight
Dapsone	With trimethoprim or chloroquine for prophylaxis of resistant strains	Slight

the introduction of synthetic antimalarials is now being used for the treatment of chloroquine resistant infections in Asia. Sulfonamides and sulfones in combination with trimethoprim can be used for treatment and prophylaxis respectively (100). In Africa, serious drug resistance to chloroquine has not developed although the dosage required for prophylaxis has been raised to two tablets weekly (172). Chloroquine or amodiaquine are the drugs of choice for treatment. Some experts prefer to use a different drug, pyrimethamine, for prophylaxis while others rely on chloroquine for both treatment and prophylaxis, see Table V.

Of the drugs used in the treatment or prophylaxis of malaria, the 8-aminoquinoline, primaquine, is the most active in producing hemolysis in individuals with G-6-P D deficiency (76). While normal individuals can be given 30 mg. daily for a week without ill effect this schedule must be modified for persons with known or suspected enzyme deficiency. In such persons it is safe to give 45 mg. once weekly for eight weeks and this treatment is still effective against the secondary exoerythrocytic cycle of P. vivax (3).

TABLE V
SCHEDULE OF DOSAGE FOR CHLOROQUINE: TABLETS*

Age years	Prophylaxis		Treatment†	
	immunes	*non-immunes*	*immunes*	*non-immunes*
Under 1	$\frac{1}{4}$	$\frac{1}{4}$	$\frac{1}{2}$	1
1 to 3	$\frac{1}{4}$	$\frac{1}{2}$	1	2
3 to 6	$\frac{3}{8}$	$\frac{3}{4}$	$\frac{3}{2}$	3
6 to 9	$\frac{1}{2}$	1	2	4
9 to 12	$\frac{3}{4}$	$\frac{3}{2}$	3	6
Over 12	1	2	4	8
Maximum	$\frac{3}{2}$	3	6	12

* Each tablet contains 150 mg. base; total weight if sulfate is 200 mg., if phosphate 250 mg.

† These doses are for oral administration, the prophylactic dose being given once a week and the therapeutic dose over a period of 24 to 72 hours. When parenteral treatment is necessary the dose should not exceed 5 mg. per kg. body weight, at 8 hour intervals.

V : The Spleen

DURING fetal life, the spleen is one of the principal sites of red cell formation. Although this function is lost in later life, the spleen continues to produce lymphocytes, monocytes and plasma cells. Furthermore, the spleen seems to exert some control over the maturation of red cells in the bone marrow. If the spleen is enlarged, it can also act as a reservoir for red cells. At all times the spleen plays a role in red cell destruction, removing from the circulation by filtration and phagocytosis the over aged, damaged and abnormal red cells, converting hemoglobin to hemosiderin and bilirubin. Apparently the spleen is also able to remove siderotic granules from abnormal red cells by the so called pitting function (18).

Perhaps the most important activity of the spleen is to protect against infections, the reticuloendothelial cells being capable of removing bacteria from the circulation. Finally, the spleen may be a site for antibody formation (149).

Nevertheless, the individual whose spleen is removed, has only a slightly increased susceptibility to infection. With respect to bacterial infections, this hazard may last for a year or two but with respect to malaria it is a more permanent disability. Furthermore, after removal of the spleen, the red cells tend to become flatter in shape with nuclear fragments and occasional protuberances (34).

The spleen has a capsule containing smooth muscle and connecting trabeculae, a vascular system with connecting sinusoids, and a lymphoid system with discrete collections of cells called the Malpighian corpuscles. Most of the blood passes through the spleen rapidly, but a small fraction is trapped and passes slowly (65).

Splenomegaly is sometimes associated with vascular diseases, especially chronic congestive splenomegaly or Banti's syndrome. Enlargement of the spleen is also caused by certain tropical infections, leishmaniasis, schistosomiasis as well as malaria (153). The spleen is also enlarged in certain malignant diseases and lipoidoses.

Splenic enlargement may also be associated with increased red cell destruction or extramedullary blood formation. Increased erythropoesis causes an early and rapid uptake of radio-active iron while excessive sequestration and destruction of red cells causes an exaggerated late uptake of radio-active iron (148).

Because of its propensity to destroy abnormal red cells, the spleen is especially likely to become enlarged in diseases characterized by the production of abnormal red cells. If the shape of the red cells is abnormal as in hereditary spherocytosis or marked ovalocytosis, or if there is a severe abnormality in the enzyme system as in non-spherocytic hemo-lytic anemias, or if the immune reactions of the red cells are abnormal as in the auto-immune hemolytic anemias, the spleen has increased size and activity (34). Thus, the spleen shows pathological changes in the abnormal hemoglobin diseases, thalassemia and combinations of these two hereditary abnormalities of the red cell, see Table VI.

TABLE VI

THE SPLEEN IN ABNORMAL HEMOGLOBIN DISEASES IN AFRICA

Disease	Size of spleen		Hypersplenism	Siderofibrosis
	Children	Adults		
Sickle cell trait	Normal	Normal	None	None
Hemoglobin C trait	Normal	Normal	None	None
Thalessemia trait	Enlarged	Enlarged	None	None
Sickle cell anemia	Enlarged	Atrophic*	Yes	Yes
Sickle cell hemoglobin C disease	Enlarged	Enlarged	None	Slight
Sickle cell thalassemia	Enlarged	Enlarged	Yes	Slight
Thalassemia	Enlarged	Enlarged	Yes	Moderate
Hemoglobin CC	Enlarged	Enlarged	None	None

* Splenic enlargement may persist into adult life in areas where malaria is preva-lent, see Table VII.

The enlarged spleen is more susceptible to infarction and rupture than the normal spleen. Furthermore, removal of an enlarged spleen, particularly if it is over active may improve the clinical picture in thalassemia and sickle cell anemia (154).

In sickle cell anemia and sickle cell hemoglobin C disease, as observed in children in malarial areas, there is an increasing incidence of splenomegaly with age, see New Cases in Table VII (57). However, with the institution of malaria chemoprophylaxis this trend is reversed in sickle cell anemia, see Protected Cases in Table VII. The absence of malaria or the institution of malaria chemoprophylaxis does not reverse the trend of splenomegaly in sickle cell hemoglobin C disease or thalassemia. Apparently the reduction in size of the spleen in sickle cell anemia is in part the result of repeated infarction. In sickle cell

TABLE VII

COMPARISON OF INCIDENCE OF SPLENOMEGALY IN SICKLE CELL
ANEMIA IN RELATION TO AGE IN NEW CASES AND CHILDREN
PROTECTED FROM MALARIA FOR ONE YEAR*

Age in years	New cases		Protected cases	
	Number	% Splenomegaly	Number	% Splenomegaly
2	41	36	4	25
2–4	26	65	20	35
4–6	22	73	22	27
6–8	14	78	11	36
8–10+	17	65	15	7
TOTAL	120	60	72	26

* From Hendrickse in *Abnormal Haemoglobins in Africa*.

thalassemia, some cases show persistent splenomegaly and others splenic atrophy.

With exposure to decreased atmospheric pressure, as in high altitude flight in non-pressurized airplanes, infarction of the spleen may occur in individuals with sickle cell trait as well as in sickle cell anemia and sickle cell hemoglobin C disease (74).

In sickle cell anemia, the rate of red cell destruction by the spleen varies from one patient to another. When the spleen is small, the liver may be a more important site for phagocytic removal of red cells as depicted in Figure XIII, where the average half life of the red cells was 9 days and the ratio of radio-activity of the spleen to the liver was less than unity (55). On the other hand, in a patient with an average red cell half life of less than 5 days, the ratio of radio-activity of the spleen to the liver exceeded 3 by the tenth day, see Figure XIV.

Some of the enlarged spleens, in sickle cell anemia and sickle cell thalassemia, even in non-malarial areas, become over active and remove normal as well as abnormal red cells from the circulation. In such cases there is neutropenia and thrombocytopenia as well as anemia. This condition, known as hypersplenism, may also occur in individuals with a normal hemoglobin pattern who have had repeated attacks of malaria (153). In hypersplenism there is an increase in the fraction of blood which takes thirty minutes rather than thirty seconds to traverse the spleen (66). During the prolonged sojourn in the spleen, at a reduced oxygen saturation there may be an aggravation of the sickling process. Figure XV depicts a 10 year old child with sickle cell thalassemia, huge spleen, and hypersplenism. Splenectomy was performed to assist in the

CB 20 years spleen not felt

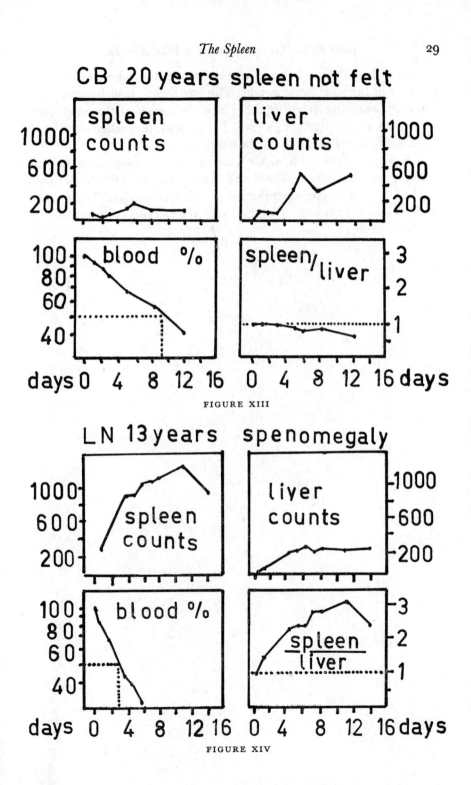

FIGURE XIII

LN 13 years spenomegaly

FIGURE XIV

control of hemolytic crises and when removed the spleen weighed 10 per cent of the total body weight. The boy had to lean backwards to counterbalance the weight of the spleen. Following splenectomy there were no more hemolytic crises (89). The patient succumbed some years later as the result of a salmonella infection.

Some patients with sickle cell anemia develop siderofibrotic nodules in the spleen. These are similar to the "Gandy-Gamma bodies" of spherocytic anemia and portal hypertension. When these nodules contain calcium as well as iron, the spleen becomes visible in the x-ray (128).

VI : Inheritance and Distribution of Hemoglobinopathies

THE TRANSMISSION of hereditary abnormalities is effected by the chromosomes. The ordinary chromosomes or autosomes are formed from two strands, one derived from the ovum and the other from the sperm. The strand of the sex chromosome of the male is shorter than that of the female so that some of the characteristics of the male are determined solely by the strand inherited from the ovum, sex-linked inheritance.

The hereditary elements or genes are arranged in a linear fashion along the length of the chromosome. The number on each chromosome is very large. The gene responsible for a given characteristic has a fixed location on the chromosome, and the analogous gene which may alter that characteristic occurs at the same location on the chromosome. Pairs of genes are called alleles and the characteristics are said to be allelic.

Apparently most of the beta chain hemoglobin abnormalities such as hemoglobins S, C, E, D persistent F hemoglobin and beta thalassemia are allelic and four hemoglobins are found only in those rare instances when there is both an alpha and beta chain mutation in the same individual (63).

A single altered gene paired with a normal allele may be strong enough to determine the bodily characteristic involved. In such instances, the altered gene is said to be dominant. In other cases, the body character or phenotype does not show any effect from the altered gene so that the hereditary pattern or genotype is concealed. Such genes are said to be recessive and do not come to light unless a pair of recessive genes are inherited. The hemoglobinopathies, in general, occupy an intermediate position, the altered gene being neither dominant nor recessive but codominant or intermediate. In this type of inheritance, both the normal and the abnormal gene contribute to the phenotype. In such cases the inheritance is heterozygous and the condition is known as trait. If two abnormal genes are inherited, the condition is known as homozygous and there is disease (126). There is an interesting relationship between the percentage of individuals showing the trait and the disease, see Table VIII. The frequency of the disease is proportional to the square of the frequency of the trait.

TABLE VIII

FREQUENCY OF THE GENE, HETEROZYGOUS AND HOMOZYGOUS*

Frequency of the gene S hemoglobin	Frequency of the trait for sickle cell	Frequency of the disease sickle cell anemia	Ratio of disease to trait
%	%	%	%
1	1·98	0·01	0·5
2	3·92	0·04	1·0
5	9·5	0·25	2·5
10	18	1	5·5
20	32	4	12·5
30	42	9	21·5
40	48	16	33·3
50	50	25	50·0

* The same figures hold for hemoglobin C, D, E, etc. and for beta thalassemia.

The genes contain desoxyribonucleic acid or DNA and the order of the four different bases in this molecule determines the type of amino acid to be synthesized in the chain of the protein. However, the message to the protein forming ribosome is transmitted by ribosenucleic acid RNA, whose arrangement of bases is determined by the DNA, see Table IX (81). In West Africa the common genotypes are AA, AS, AC,

TABLE IX

THE GENETIC CODE FOR COMMON ABNORMAL HEMOGLOBINS

Hemoglobin	Chain involved	Number of the amino acid	Code of bases on the RNA*	Amino acid produced
A	beta	6	UAG	Glutamic
A	beta	26	UAG	Glutamic
A	beta	121	UAG	Glutamic
S	beta	6	UUG	Valine
C	beta	6	UAA	Lysine
D$_{Punjab}$	beta	121	UCG	Glutamine
E	beta	26	UAA	Lysine

* A = adeneine, G = Guanine, C = cytosine and U = uracil.

Ath, SC, SS, CC and Sth. The rare genotypes are Cth and thth, where th stands for beta thalassemia, AO, AG and AF, where F stands for persistent fetal hemoglobin.

   If one parent has sickle cell trait and the other a normal hemoglobin pattern, half the children will have a normal hemoglobin pattern and half will inherit the trait. But when both parents have sickle cell trait, one quarter will inherit sickle cell anemia, see Table X. Although

TABLE X

INHERITANCE OF S HEMOGLOBIN

Parents		Children		
Mother	*Father*	*AA* %	*AS* %	*SS* %
AA	AA	100	0	0
AS AA	AA AS	50	50	0
AS	AS	25	50	25
SS AA	AA SS	0	100	0
SS AS	AS SS	0	50	50
SS	SS	0	0	100

the statistics predict these ratios, in any particular family, all of the children may be normal, or all may have sickle cell anemia just as in some large families all the children are female and in others all male.

In many parts of Africa, the incidence of sickle cell trait is twenty per cent. Table XI shows that in the next generation there will be a

TABLE XI

INHERITANCE OF S HEMOGLOBIN
IN A POPULATION WITH 20 PER CENT TRAIT

Parents				Progeny		
Maternal pattern	%	*Paternal pattern*	%	*AA* %	*AS* %	*SS* %
		AA	80	64	0	0
AA	80					
		AS	20	8	8	0
		AA	80	8	8	0
AS	20					
		AS	20	1	2	1
TOTAL				81	18	1

reduction in the incidence of trait due to the combination of some genes to form sickle cell anemia. Since the survival and reproduction rate for sickle cell anemia is low there will be a gradual reduction in the incidence of sickle cell trait. However, the trait will persist and increase in highly malarial areas where the child with sickle cell trait has a better chance of surviving than the child with normal hemoglobin (92).

There are some parts of Africa where there is a ten per cent incidence of sickle cell hemoglobin C trait and a twenty per cent incidence of sickle cell trait. Under these conditions, Table XII, two per

TABLE XII

INHERITANCE OF S AND C HEMOGLOBINS
IN A POPULATION WITH S AND C TRAITS

Parents				Progeny					
Maternal		Paternal		AA	AS	AC	SC	SS	CC
pat.	%	pat.	%	%	%	%	%	%	%
AA	70	AA	70	49					
		AS	20	7	7				
		AC	10	3½		3½			
AS	20	AA	70	7	7				
		AS	20	1	2			1	
		AC	10	½	½	½	½		
AC	10	AA	70	3½		3½			
		AS	20	½	½	½	½		
		AC	10	¼		½			¼
TOTAL				72¼	17	8½	1	1	¼

cent of the children will be born with sickle cell disease, half with sickle cell anemia and half with sickle cell hemoglobin C disease. In addition there will be ¼ per cent of homozygous hemoglobin C disease (129).

The world wide distribution of common abnormal hemoglobin diseases, thalassemia and G-6-P D deficiency is illustrated in Figure XVI. The areas involved have all been affected by falciparum malaria for centuries, in fact, thousands of years. Of course the descendants of these people who have migrated or have been forced to migrate to the Americas have brought these genetic abnormalities with them. It is thought that S hemoglobin probably originated in the Middle East and was carried eastward to India and westward to Africa whence it spread throughout the tropical belt (81).

The distribution of S hemoglobin in Africa is shown in Figure XVII. The numbers given represent country averages and there are wide fluctuations within each country. The northern and southern extremes of the African continent are almost free of sickle hemoglobin. The distribution of hemoglobin C is much more limited, see Figure XVIII. This abnormality is present in greatest concentration in Upper Volta and northern Ghana and Togo. The mutation may have arisen long after the S mutation and in Africa rather than Asia. The distribution of beta thalassemia in Africa is patchy and not well known but some estimates are given in Figure XIX (92) (126).

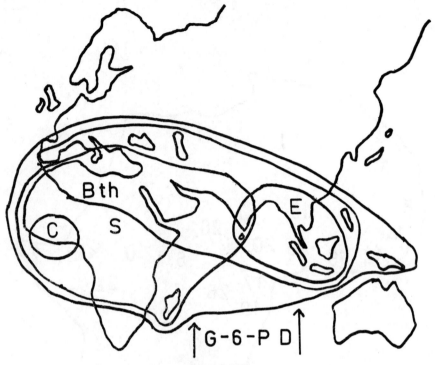

FIGURE XVI
World distribution

The world wide distribution of G-6-P D deficiency, Figure XVI, covers the same area as the abnormal hemoglobins plus beta thalassemia (127). However, the type of G-6-P D deficiency in Africa is different from the type observed in the Mediterranean and Asia (15). The distribution of G-6-P D deficiency in Africa is shown in Figure XX. Here, the area involved corresponds with the distribution of abnormal hemoglobins and beta thalassemia.

Population-wise, there is a good correlation between the incidence of sickle cell hemoglobin and G-6-P D deficiency in Africa, between the incidence of sickle cell hemoglobin and G-6-P D deficiency in Greece, and between beta thalassemia and G-6-P D deficiency in Sardinia. This correlation has been explained on the basis that malaria is the common denominator responsible for the maintenance of a high level of the three abnormalities (92). On the other hand, there is a negative correlation between S and C hemoglobins in Africa and a negative correlation between S hemoglobin and thalassemia in Greece. This can be explained

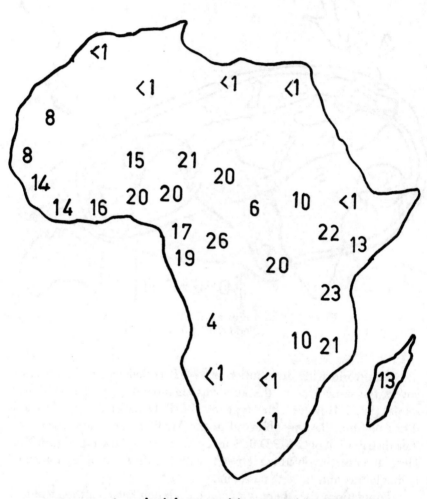

per cent sickle cell trait (WHO)

FIGURE XVII

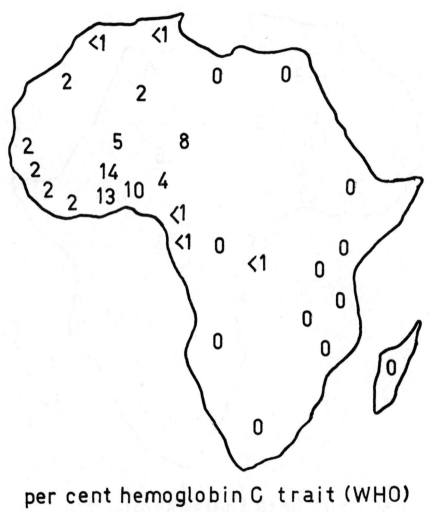

per cent hemoglobin C trait (WHO)

FIGURE XVIII

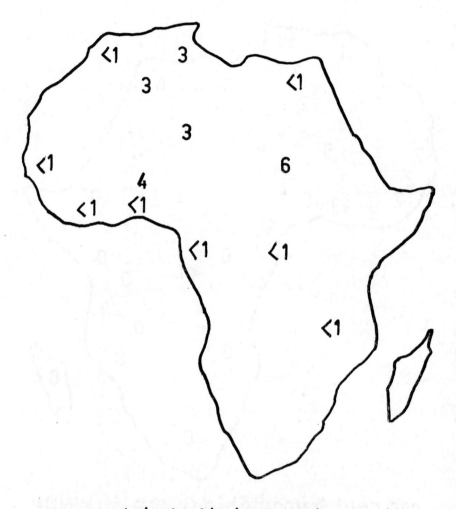

per cent beta thalassemia trait
(WHO)

FIGURE XIX

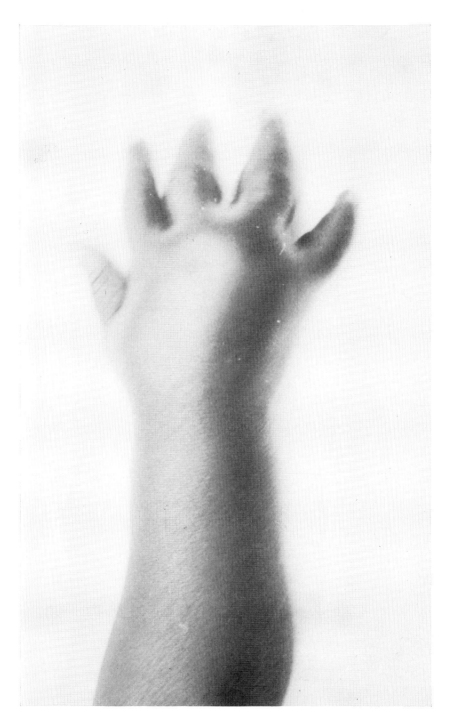

FIGURE XXIV

Hand-foot syndrome

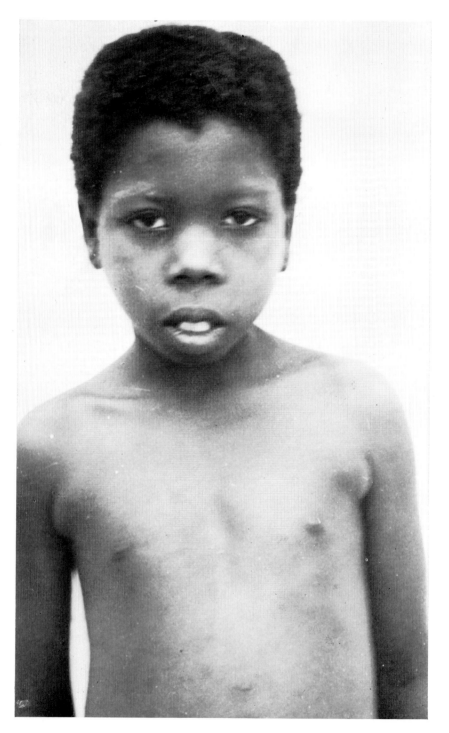

FIGURE XXV

Characteristic fascies with prominent upper teeth

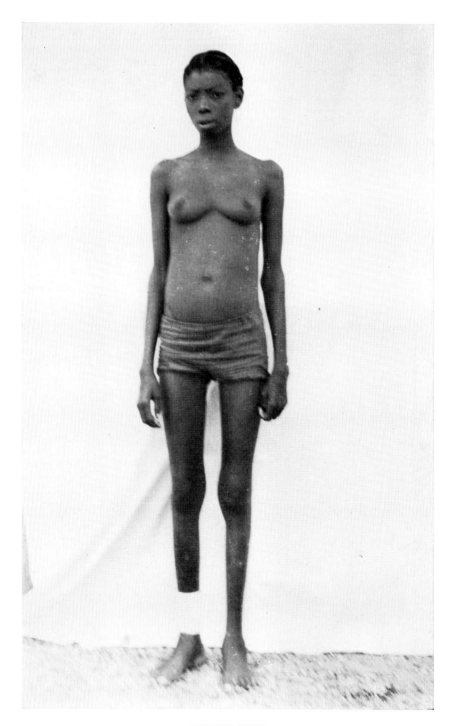

FIGURE XXVI

Asthenic habitus in sickle cell thalassemia

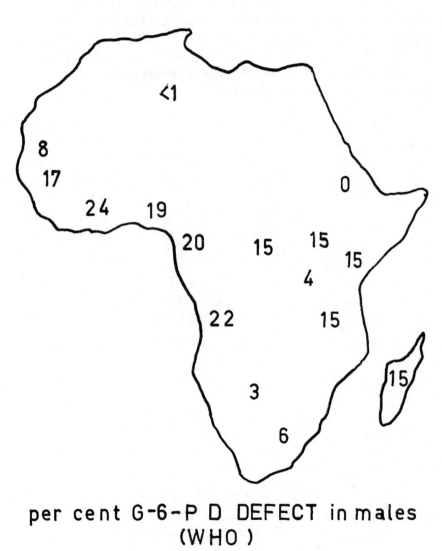

per cent G-6-P D DEFECT in males
(WHO)

FIGURE XX

by the fact that the two characteristics are allelic and the individual with both abnormalities has a reduced biological fitness.

It is interesting to note that the American Negroes who came originally from West Africa have a ten per cent incidence of sickle cell trait and an eleven per cent incidence of G-6-P D defect (126). The reduction in the incidence of sickle cell trait is in a small part due to admixture with the caucasian race and to a larger extent due to the low biological fitness of sickle cell anemia.

VII : The Chemistry and Physiology
of Sickling

IN S HEMOGLOBIN the sixth amino acid of the beta chains, namely glutamic acid, has been replaced by valine with the loss of one electron or a positive gain of one electric charge in each beta chain. The resultant decrease in the speed of migration of S hemoglobin in an electric current has been illustrated. Nevertheless, when fully oxygenated, S hemoglobin has almost the same physical properties as normal hemoglobin.

However, when S hemoglobin is reduced, it tends to come out of solution in the form of tactoids or spindle shaped microcrystals, forming a gel. This process distorts the shape of the red cells which then become susceptible to magnetic force and will orient perpendicular to the lines of force, see Figure XXI (105).

The formation of these micro-crystals has been explained on the basis that the valine at position 6 is attracted by the valine at position 1 allowing a peptide link to form between the valine at position 1 and the threonine at position 4, see Figure XXII (105).

The presence of a hydrophobic union is consistent with the observation that gels composed of reduced S hemoglobin can be made to go back in solution with huge pressure or very low temperature. The chemical bonds that are formed permit a linear stacking of the hemoglobin molecules. Several such strands, six, may twist about a central core to form a sort of hollow "microtubule". Such structures have been seen in the electron microphotographs (105) and may account for the rotation of polarized light and birefringence of the gel (53).

The microcrystals are responsible for the distortion in shape of red cells containing reduced S hemoglobin. In the early stages of sickling the red cell becomes elongated or oat shaped. Then protuberances appear or a holly leaf appearance is created, Figure VIII. As deoxygenation proceeds, the cell sends out long filaments. Up to a certain stage the process can be reversed if the oxygen tension is raised. But after the filaments are formed, reversal leads to a loss of substance and damage to the membrane.

The most important factor affecting the sickling tendency is the partial pressure of oxygen or the oxygen saturation of the hemoglobin.

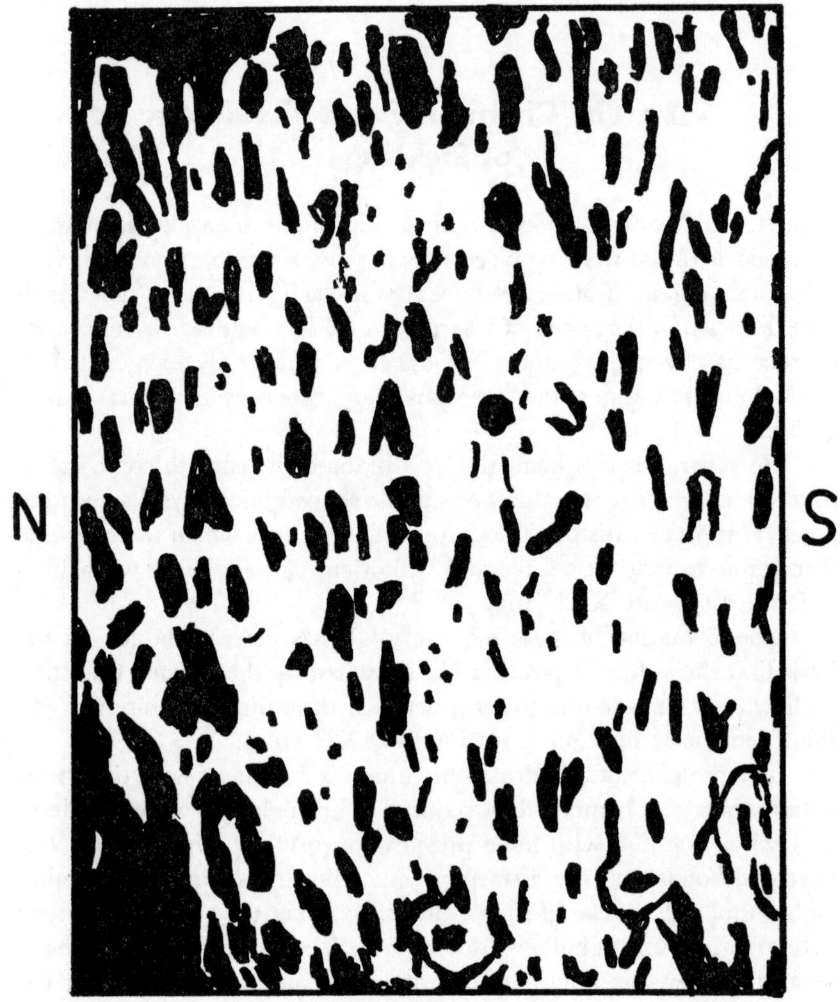

FIGURE XXI
Magnetically oriented sickled erythrocytes
From Murayama, 1966

This can be controlled during *in vitro* experiments, see Figure XXIII (50). Similar changes can be brought about *in vivo* by reducing the oxygen content of inspired air or by reducing the atmospheric pressure. This happens during high altitude flight in non-pressurized planes causing splenic infarct in individuals with sickle cell trait or disease (151).

The next most important factor affecting the sickling of red cells is

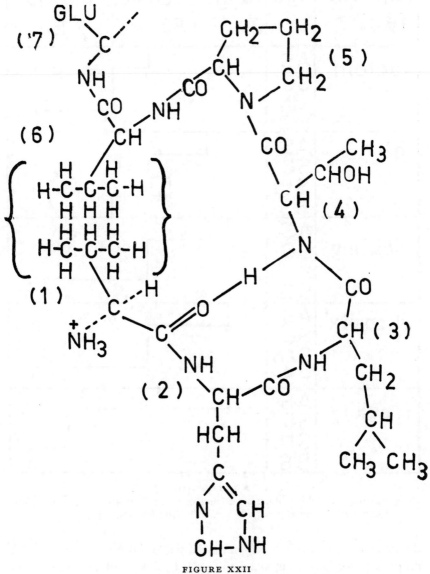

FIGURE XXII
Chemical bonding at the end of the beta S chain
From Murayama, 1966

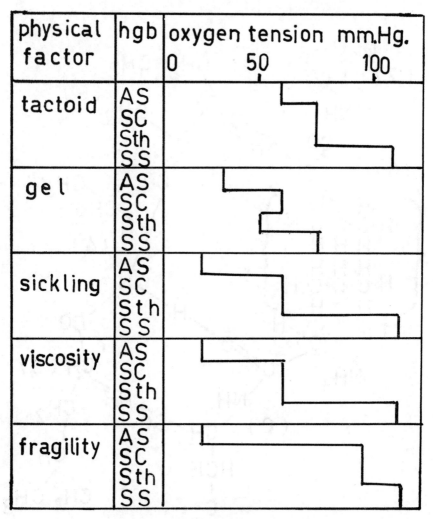

FIGURE XXIII

Oxygen tensions at which biophysical changes occur in sickle sell disease. (From Griggs, R. C. and Harris, J. W., *A.M.A. Arch. Int. Med.* **97**:315, 1956)

the percentage of sickle hemoglobin. In sickle cell trait there is a wide range of percentage from 20 to 50 (106). In sickle cell anemia the percentage varies rom 80 to 99 depending on the amount of F hemoglobin that is present. In sickle cell thalassemia there is an even wider range of variation due to the presence of A and F hemoglobins.

It is important to note that it is not only the percentage of S that is responsible for the tendency to sickle but also the nature of the other hemoglobin that makes up the total. The degree to which the other hemoglobin tends to crystallize with S hemoglobin is called its reactivity. Of all the hemoglobins, C is the most reactive so that a person with S and C hemoglobins has sickle cell disease. On the other hand, F hemoglobin is the least reactive so that a small percentage of F will be more effective than a moderate amount of A in reducing the tendency towards sickling (65). Listing the common hemoglobins in terms of their ability to alleviate sickling one gets the series F, A, D, C (81).

In addition to the percentage of S hemoglobin and the nature of the admixed hemoglobin and the oxygen tension, there is the time required for deoxygenation. The time required for sickling is less than half a minute (69) but deoxygenation proceeds more slowly. The loss of oxygen is due almost entirely to consumption by the body tissues. But blood that stagnates in the spleen or bone marrow may loose some oxygen through consumption by formed elements, leukocytes or reticulocytes (89A). This latter phenomenon explains the sickling which takes place in sealed preparations to which no reducing agent has been added.

Other factors which may affect sickling are the hydrogen ion concentration, osmotic pressure and temperature. A high hydrogen ion concentration or low pH may accelerate sickling because it facilitates deoxygenation of blood. *In vivo* sickling crises have been produced by the administration of large amounts of ammonium chloride (10). Increased osmotic pressure also favours sickling (122) and this may account for the vulnerability of the kidney to capillary thromboses in sickle states. Very low temperatures delay sickling (105), in fever the increased oxygen consumption accelerates the sickling process (11).

Anesthesia may initiate sickling because of a reduction in oxygen saturation of the blood, because of metabolic acidosis, or because of stasis of the circulation. Pregnancy and delivery may also induce sickling for similar reasons.

It is thought that the painful crises in sickle cell disease are the result of capillary thromboses. Sometimes the thrombosis leads to infarction. The sickling and the resultant thrombosis may be considered to be due to a vicious cycle involving stasis, deoxygenation, increased carbon dioxide content and hydrogen ion concentration, increased viscosity and finally mechanical fragility and clumping of sickled cells. Any one of the above mentioned factors may initiate or aggravate the process (53).

Sensitivity to oxygen deprivation is greatest in sickle cell anemia and least in sickle cell trait (50) Sickle cell hemoglobin C disease occupies an intermediate position. But in sickle cell hemoglobin C disease, the presence of a normal or almost normal hemoglobin level instead of an anemia makes for a much greater viscosity so that patients with sickle cell hemoglobin C disease are especially susceptible to thromboses and infarction. Sickle cell thalassemia occupies a position between sickle cell anemia and sickle cell hemoglobin C disease (53) and the sensitivity to oxygen deprivation is an inverse function of the level of fetal hemoglobin (65). *In vitro* comparisons of sensitivity to oxygen deprivation are illustrated in Figure XXIII which gives the percentage of sickle cells, increase in viscosity and mechanical fragility as well as tactoid and gel formation (50).

Sickle cell disease is characterized not only by a tendency to thrombotic episodes, but also by a greatly increased rate of production and destruction of red cells with an equilibrium at a lower hemoglobin level than in normal subjects. This phenomenon produces an increased percentage of nucleated red cells and reticulocytes, an increased level of serum bilirubin, and an expansion in the size of the bone marrow cavities to accommodate the erythropoetic tissue. The latter may lead to thinning of the cortex of the long bones and expansion of the diploic spaces of the skull which is especially pronounced in sickle cell anemia and sickle cell thalassemia (128). In sickle cell hemoglobin C and sickle cell hemoglobin D diseases the half life of the red cells is not so greatly shortened, see Table XIV, and the hemoglobin level may reach normal (130).

The high rate of red cell destruction in sickle cell anemia is only in part due to removal of sickled cells from the circulation. As a matter of fact, the spleen removes cells containing abnormal hemoglobin even in the absence of sickling as in homozygous hemoglobin C or E diseases. Also, hemolytic episodes are not uncommon in children and pregnant women when there are no thrombotic episodes. Enlargement of the spleen, even in the absence of hypersplenism, may be associated with an increased rate of red cell destruction and pooling of the blood. Removal of the enlarged spleen may lead to a prolongation of the half life of the red cells, see Table XIII (154).

Very short red cell survival rates have been described in cases of sickle cell anemia and megaloblastic erythropoesis associated with deficiency of folic acid (167). Whether the folic acid deficiency is the cause or the result of the extremely short red cell survival is not clear but the survival studies were carried out after the administration of folic acid, and long term treatment included anti-malarials as well as folic acid.

TABLE XIII

RED CELL HALF LIFE IN RELATION TO
HEMOGLOBIN PATTERN AND SPLEEN SIZE

Hemoglobin	Number of cases	Size of spleen	Red cell half life (days)	Same after splenectomy (days)
AA†	—	0	30	—
SC†	7	0 to 4t	16	—
SS†	7	0	10	—
SS*	4	0	8	—
SS†	5	1 to 4t	4·0	11
SS*	7	2 to 4t	4·5	—

*From Hathorn and Lewis.   † From Sprague and Paterson.

VIII : Diagnosis of Sickle Cell States

SICKLE cell trait is not a disease. For this and other reasons it is almost impossible to make a clinical distinction between a person with normal hemoglobin and one with sickle cell trait. The only clues to the existence of sickle cell trait are idiopathic hematuria and infarction following airplane flight.

On the other hand, it is often possible to make a clinical diagnosis of sickle cell disease on the basis of the history and physical findings, see Table XIV. In fact, it is sometimes possible to distinguish between sickle cell anemia and sickle cell hemoglobin C disease, as the former has a greater degree of anemia and jaundice while the latter is characterized by a more normal hemoglobin level and the persistence of splenomegaly (150). However, the clinical diagnosis should be checked by laboratory examinations, see Table XV.

In infants, sickle cell disease may be suspected when there is marked pallor, jaundice, failure to thrive, and repeated or severe infections. But it is possible to confuse malnutrition and chronic infection with sickle cell disease unless there is an acute hemolytic crisis or hand foot syndrome (166). In this syndrome there is painful swelling of the fingers or toes and often the dorsum of the hand or the entire foot, see Figure XXIV. These infants often have fever, hepatomegaly and splenomegaly. Cardiac murmurs, cardiomegaly and tachycardia may be present (107). Some infants show frontal bossing and a square shaped head, see Figure XXV.

In older children, the diagnosis of sickle cell disease should be suspected again when there is pallor, jaundice, failure to thrive and recurrent infections. Hemolytic crises and hand foot syndrome are not as common as during infancy but periodic attacks of rheumatic pain and occasional abdominal crises are characteristic. As in infants, splenomegaly and hepatomegaly are common. As the child grows there is a tendency to attain a slender habitus with long tapering fingers, see Figure XXVI. Such children look younger than the stated age. A few cases develop prominent upper incisor teeth with malocclusion as in Cooley's anemia (89), see Figure XXV. Periodic attacks of jaundice are common, especially in those patients who also have a deficiency in G-6-P D (87). The family history helps in making a diagnosis as

TABLE XIV

CLINICAL FINDINGS IN SICKLE CELL DISEASE ACCORDING TO AGE*

Clinical finding	Infants	Children	Adults
Pallor	+	+	+
Jaundice	+	+	+
Cardiac enlargement	+	+	+
Cardiac murmurs	+	+	+
Tachycardia	+	+	+
Dyspnoea	+	+	+
Fever	+	+	+
Hepatomegaly	+	+	+
Osteomyelitis	+	+	+
Splenomegaly	+	+	−
Lympadenopathy	+	+	−
Recurrent infections	+	+	−
Hand foot syndrome	+	−	−
Hemolytic crises	+	−	−
Failure to thrive	+	−	−
Frontal bossing	+	−	−
Abdominal crises	−	+	−
Epistaxis	−	+	−
Aplastic crises	−	+	−
Cutaneous ulcers	−	+	+
Slender habitus	−	+	+
Fatiguability	−	+	+
Rheumatic pains	−	+	+
Painful crises	−	+	+
Aseptic bone necrosis	−	+	+
Hematuria	−	+	+
Priapism	−	+	+
Delayed development	−	+	+
Retinal detachment	−	−	+
Vitreous hemorrhage	−	−	+
Frequent abortions	−	−	+

* An approximate guide, not all signs and symptoms are present and occasionally may occur at any age.

siblings may suffer from the same disease which often ends fatally between the age of six months and two years. In older children, sickle cell hemoglobin C disease may be suspected when there are frequent attacks of rheumatic pains but no anemia or jaundice.

In adults, a clinical diagnosis of sickle cell disease may be entertained when there is pallor, icterus, episodes of severe pain and a history of chronic rheumatic pains since childhood. Splenomegaly persisting into adult life is more common in sickle cell hemoglobin C disease than sickle cell anemia. Women with sickle cell anemia rarely have more than one or two children and give a history of having had spontaneous abortions (71). A limp due to aseptic necrosis of the head of the femur (32) or sudden loss of vision in one eye from vitreous hemorrhage (104) should evoke suspicion of sickle cell disease and these events are more likely to be seen in sickle cell hemoglobin C disease than in sickle cell anemia (150). However, such events are quite common in sickle cell anemia in Jamaica where the disease seems to pursue a more benign course (144).

Despite the many signs and symptoms associated with sickle cell disease, the diagnosis is sometimes made by routine blood examination when the individual is asymptomatic or suffering from some other ailment. The diagnosis is sometimes made by an alert ophthalmologist (90), dentist or radiologist (128).

The simplest laboratory procedure involved in the diagnosis of sickle cell states is the sickle test, which determines the presence or absence of S hemoglobin but does not distinguish between sickle cell trait and sickle cell disease (142). When a drop of freshly prepared solution of sodium metabisulfite is added to a drop of blood and the preparation is observed for an hour, a negative test rules out the possibility of sickle cell trait or sickle cell disease except in cord blood and the first months of life. If the test is carried out without the addition of a reducing agent and the preparation is sealed and kept in an incubator for 24 hours, the speed of sickling and the type of sickled cell gives a clue as to whether the individual has sickle cell trait or sickle cell disease (34). The absence of anemia does not rule out sickle cell hemoglobin C disease or sickle cell trait but is not compatible with sickle cell anemia. The presence of anemia is of no diagnostic significance. The definitive diagnosis is made by means of electrophoretic analysis (115).

In a busy hospital it is possible to reduce the number of specimens that have to be examined by electrophoresis if a careful sickling test is done first and only the positive specimens subjected to analysis by electrophoresis. If this order of procedure is established, the presence of hemoglobin C trait, which is unimportant, and the diagnosis of homozygous hemoglobin C disease, which is rare in most parts of Africa, will be missed. The electrophoretic analysis gives a precise differentiation between sickle cell trait, sickle cell anemia and sickle cell hemoglobin C disease. It does not usually distinguish between sickle cell anemia, sickle cell hemoglobin D disease and sickle cell thalassemia. Additional tests are required to establish a diagnosis of these rare conditions as well as sickle cell hemoglobin with high fetal hemoglobin gene, see Table XV (81).

TABLE XV

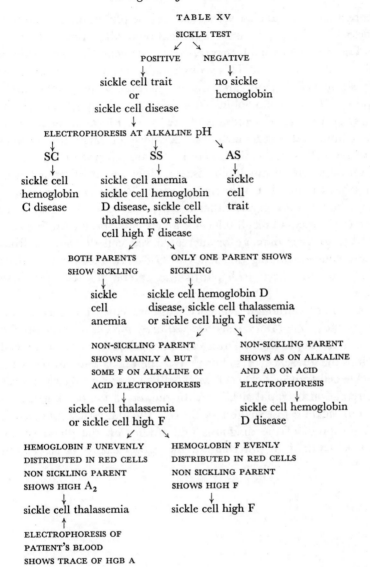

SICKLE TEST

POSITIVE   NEGATIVE

sickle cell trait
or
sickle cell disease

no sickle
hemoglobin

ELECTROPHORESIS AT ALKALINE pH

SC   SS   AS

sickle cell
hemoglobin
C disease

sickle cell anemia
sickle cell hemoglobin
D disease, sickle cell
thalassemia or sickle
cell high F disease

sickle
cell
trait

BOTH PARENTS   ONLY ONE PARENT SHOWS
SHOW SICKLING   SICKLING

sickle
cell
anemia

sickle cell hemoglobin D
disease, sickle cell thalassemia
or sickle cell high F disease

NON-SICKLING PARENT
SHOWS MAINLY A BUT
SOME F ON ALKALINE or
ACID ELECTROPHORESIS

NON-SICKLING PARENT
SHOWS AS ON ALKALINE
AND AD ON ACID
ELECTROPHORESIS

sickle cell thalassemia
or sickle cell high F

sickle cell hemoglobin
D disease

HEMOGLOBIN F UNEVENLY
DISTRIBUTED IN RED CELLS
NON SICKLING PARENT
SHOWS HIGH A_2

HEMOGLOBIN F EVENLY
DISTRIBUTED IN RED CELLS
NON SICKLING PARENT
SHOWS HIGH F

sickle cell thalassemia

sickle cell high F

ELECTROPHORESIS OF
PATIENT'S BLOOD
SHOWS TRACE OF HGB A

If the patient's electrophoresis shows SS hemoglobin pattern, the diagnosis of sickle cell hemoglobin D disease may be suspected when one of the parents shows the electrophoretic pattern of sickle cell trait yet there is no sickling. The diagnosis of sickle cell thalassemia may be suspected when one of the parents shows no evidence of S hemoglobin by electrophoresis or sickling test.

There are certain ancillary tests that are helpful in the diagnosis of sickle states (62). One of these is the estimation of alkali resistant hemoglobin. The result is usually expressed as per cent fetal hemoglobin out of the total hemoglobin. This is often higher than the normal, $\frac{1}{2}$ per cent, in sickle cell anemia and sickle cell thalassemia, only rarely elevated in sickle cell hemoglobin C disease and never in sickle cell trait, except during the first few months of life (161). Elevation of the reticulocyte count and particularly the presence of large numbers of nucleated red cells suggests that there is a hemolytic anemia but is not specific for abnormal hemoglobin disease. However, it is important to be aware that the number of nucleated red cells may be so great that the usual white count suggests either marked leucocytosis or leukemia. Elevation of the serum bilirubin level is a very non-specific finding as it may be due to liver damage or increased red cell destruction from almost any cause including deficiency of G-6-P D. Sickle cell crisis is often confused with infectious hepatitis and amebic hepatitis for these reasons.

In summary, although sickle cell disease can be suspected on clinical grounds, laboratory tests are required for a sure and precise diagnosis. The simple sickling test can be used to exclude sickle cell disease but the presence of sickling and anemia is compatible with either sickle cell trait or sickle cell disease. The presence of sickled cells in the circulation or rapid sickling with the formation of filaments in the 24 hour sickling test suggest sickle cell anemia. Electrophoresis is required for proof of the diagnosis and studies on the blood of the parents are required to differentiate the rare variants of sickle cell disease.

IX : Sickle Cell Trait

THE INDIVIDUAL with sickle cell trait has inherited one gene that causes the formation of normal beta chains and normal hemoglobin, and one gene that makes S type beta chains and S hemoglobin. The proportion of normal and S hemoglobins is not equal and varies from one individual to another, see Figure XXVII (106). Apparently there

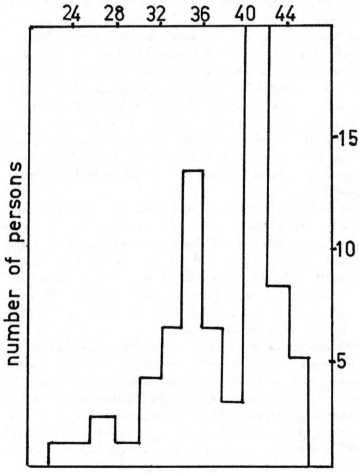

FIGURE XXVII
Proportion of S hemoglobin in sickle cell trait
Neel *et al.*, 1961

is a group of individuals with an average level of 41 per cent S hemoglobin and another group with an average of 35 per cent, although the overall range is 30 to 46 per cent.

There are a few individuals with less than 30 per cent S hemoglobin. This may be due to complicating disease such as megaloblastic anemia (56) or iron deficiency (82). Also, in alpha thalassemia, there is a reduced capacity to form normal alpha chains and this favours the formation of normal hemoglobin, and this leads to a reduction in the proportion of S hemoglobin in sickle cell trait (168), and C hemoglobin in C trait (129).

On the other hand, when an individual with sickle cell trait also inherits beta thalassemia trait there is difficulty in the formation of normal beta chains so that the blood contains mostly S hemoglobin. Such an individual has sickle cell thalassemia. As previously noted sickle cell thalassemia is a disease that rivals sickle cell anemia in severity and can be distinguished with certainty by investigation of the family.

It has been shown that the percentage of S hemoglobin is a crucial factor in determining the extent of stickling at any given oxygen tension (50). Where quantitative studies have been made among individuals with sickle cell trait who have suffered splenic infarction after airplane flight, it has been found that they had a relatively high percentage of S hemoglobin (134).

The world wide distribution of S hemoglobin has been shown in Figure XVI, the distribution in Africa in Figure XVII. A more precise estimate of the number of individuals with sickle cell trait is given in Table XVI (126). It may be seen that there are more than 28 million Africans with sickle cell trait out of a total population of 250 million. Similarly, among the 22 million Americans of African descent there are 10 per cent with sickle cell trait. In the Caribbean, Central and South America there are many more.

Although sickle cell trait may be classified as a hemoglobinopathy, it is an inherited abnormality not a disease. The red cells of individuals with sickle cell trait are almost normal unless and until the blood is deoxygenated. The number of red cells, the hemoglobin level of the blood and the volume of packed red cells are entirely normal. Even the length of red cell survival is normal (147). However, the red cells in sickle cell trait are less susceptible to osmotic hemolysis than normal red cells (53).

The biological advantage of sickle cell trait as a protection against childhood malaria has been stressed (92). It has also been claimed that

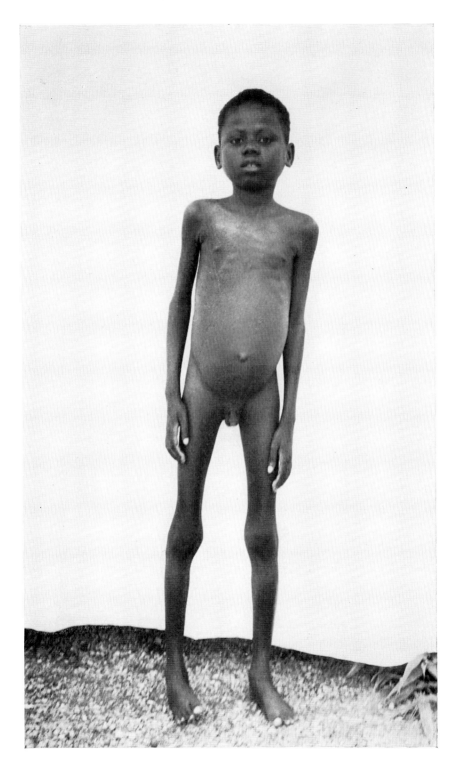

FIGURE XXVIII

Malnutrition and hepatomegaly

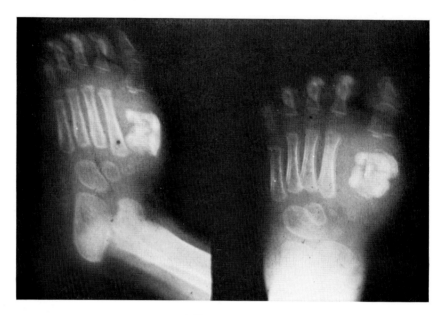

FIGURE XXXI
Bone destruction in hand-foot syndrome

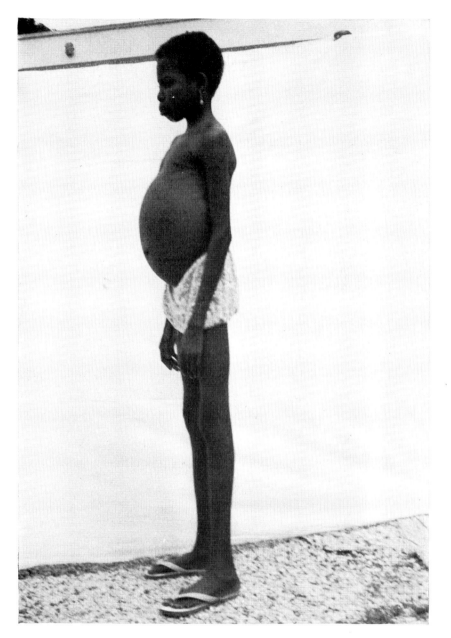

FIGURE XXXII

Hepatomegaly, splenomegaly and cardiac failure in sickle cell anemia

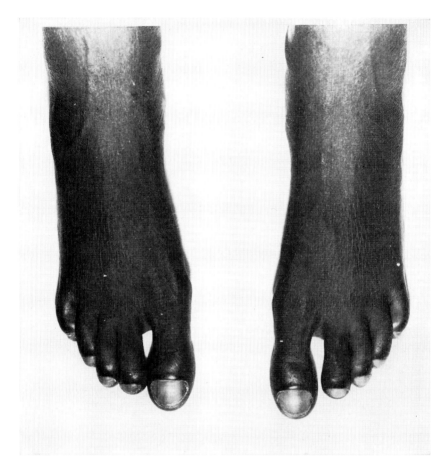

FIGURE XXXIII

Clubbing of toes in sickle cell anemia and cardiac failure

TABLE XVI

APPROXIMATE INCIDENCE OF SICKLE CELL TRAIT IN AFRICA
AND THEORETICAL NUMBER OF CASES BORN WITH
SICKLE CELL ANEMIA

Country	*Population thousands*	*Sickle cell incidence* %	*Trait number thousands*	*Sickle cell anemia thousands*
Algeria	11,600	1·5	170	—
Angola	5,100	4·3	200	2
Basutoland	—	—	—	—
Bechuanaland	—	—	—	—
Burundi	2,600	14	364	13
Cameroon	5,100	17	864	37
Central African Rep.	1,320	—	—	—
Chad	2,800	20	560	28
Congo (Brazzaville)	830	26	216	12
Congo (Kinshasa)	15,300	20	3,060	153
Dahomey	2,250	17	382	15
Equatorial Guinea	263	—	—	—
Ethiopia	2,200	—	—	—
French Somaliland	80	—	—	—
Gabon	454	19	87	4
Gambia	324	14	44	1
Ghana	7,340	16	1,140	45
Guinea	3,420	14	479	17
Ivory Coast	3,750	12	450	14
Kenya	9,100	12	1,092	33
Liberia	1,041	14	146	5
Libya	1,560	0	—	—
Madagascar	6,180	12	741	22
Malawi	3,750	—	—	—
Nigeria	55,670	20	11,130	557
Portuguese Guinea	525	10	52	1
Reunion	382	—	—	—
Rwanda	3,020	3	91	—
Senegal	3,400	8	272	5
Sierra Leone	2,190	27	610	41
Somalia	2,300	—	—	—
South Africa	17,470	—	—	—
Southwest Africa	554	—	—	—
Southern Rhodesia	4,140	10	414	10
Sudan	13,180	10	132	33
Swaziland	285	0	—	—
Togo	1,603	23	368	20
Tunisia	4,494	2	90	—
Uganda	7,190	21	1,510	79
United Arab Republic	27,960	—	—	—
Tanzania	10,315	22	2,210	129
Upper Volta	4,720	6	283	4
Zambia	3,600	15	540	20
TOTAL	254,000		28,420	1,320

sickle cell trait may increase the fertility of women in malarial areas and leads to the birth of heavier infants (135). The mechanism through which S hemoglobin protects against malaria is not clear. It is possible that the presence of the malarial parasite in the red cell leads to sickling and destruction of the cell before the parasite has a chance to mature. Such an explanation would not account for the suspected protection that is afforded by other types of abnormal hemoglobin, thalassemia and G-6-P D deficiency.

The blood traversing the capillaries adjacent to the renal tubules is subjected to a greater degree of anoxia and hemoconcentration than anywhere else in the body. This may explain why the individual with sickle cell trait is subject to microscopic hematuria and also unable to produce as concentrated a urine as normal individuals (31). A much more serious event is the appearance of gross hematuria (13). The bleeding may be so severe as to necessitate repeated transfusions. Apparently the left kidney is affected somewhat more often than the right, but in some instances when the left kidney has been removed there has been subsequent bleeding from the right (86). The blood in the renal pelvis may cause a filling defect as seen in the x-ray, and if the presence of sickling is overlooked an erroneous diagnosis may be entertained. Bacteruria and pyelonephritis in the course of pregnancy is twice as common in women with sickle cell trait as in women with a normal hemoglobin pattern (170). However, this finding must be weighed against the statistics which show that there is no difference in fertility, abortion rate, incidence of toxemia, prematurity, or perinatal mortality of infants, between mothers with sickle cell trait and those with a normal hemoglobin pattern (170).

Exposure to reduced oxygen tension in airplane flight is sometimes followed by infarction of the spleen (74) or pulmonary infarction (88). Similarly, prolonged exposure to low oxygen tension during anesthesia can cause difficulty in patients with sickle cell trait (46).

For reasons that are not clear, it appears that salmonella infections are more common in individuals with sickle cell trait than in persons with a normal hemoglobin pattern, see Table XVII (121).

Another organ that is especially susceptible to damage is the eye. Retinal hemorrhage may occur in sickle cell trait and in rare cases this may lead to retinal detachment (90). Vitreous hemorrhages which are common in sickle cell disease may also occur in sickle cell trait (104).

Priapism is yet another rare event in sickle cell trait (79). Bone lesions of sufficient severity to cause symptoms are also rare and

TABLE XVII

INCIDENCE OF SICKLE-CELL TRAIT AMONG ADMISSIONS
TO A CHILDREN'S WARD

Disease group	Total Number	Sickle cell trait Number	%
Miscellaneous	186	25	13
Pneumonia	118	18	15
Upper Respiratory Infect.	59	13	15
Diarrhoea and Vomiting	106	25	24
Poliomyelitis	26	4	15
Tuberculosis	37	8	22
Meningitis (purulent)	26	5	19
Malnutrition	77	11	14
Hookworm Anemia	30	2	7
Typhoid Fever	17	6	35
Uncomplicated Malaria	83	13	16
Cerebral Malaria	47	0	0
Blackwater Fever	6	0	0
TOTAL	818	130	16

A. B. Raper, 1956

although aseptic necrosis of the head of the femur has been described in an individual with sickle cell trait (124), it also occurs in people with a normal hemoglobin pattern (114).

However, the greatest liability of the individual with sickle cell trait is that if he marries an individual with sickle cell trait, hemoglobin C trait, or beta thalassemia trait, and has a large family, some of the children are likely to inherit sickle cell disease.

X : Types of Hemoglobinopathy

THE COMMON types of hemoglobinopathy in Africa are listed according to their genotype in Table XVIII. The list includes sickle cell trait,

TABLE XVIII

GENOTYPE OF HEMOGLOBINOPATHIES

	Gene A HGB	Gene S HGB	Gene C HGB	Gene beta thalassemia
Normal	2	0	0	0
Sickle trait	1	1	0	0
HGB C Trait	1	0	1	0
Thalassemia trait	2	0	0	1
Sickle cell anemia	0	2	0	0
Sickle cell HGB C dis.	0	1	1	0
Sickle cell thalassemia	1	1	0	1
Homozygous HGB C dis.	0	0	2	0
Thalassemia major	2	0	0	2
Hemoglobin C thalassemia	1	0	1	1

hemoglobin C trait, thalassemia trait, three types of sickle cell disease, hemoglobin C disease and thalassemia major. The three types of sickle cell disease are sickle cell anemia, sickle cell hemoglobin C disease and sickle cell thalassemia. The latter is a combination of sickle cell trait and beta thalassemia trait which produces a clinical picture similar to but sometimes less severe than sickle cell anemia, see Tables XIX and XX (168).

TABLE XIX

PHENOTYPE OF HEMOGLOBINOPATHIES

	% A	% S	% C	% F	% A_2
Normal	95–99	0	0	0–2	1–3
Sickle trait	51–73	25–46	0	0–2	1–3
HGB C trait	85–95	0	28–44	0–2	1–2
Thalassemia trait	85–95	0	0	1–10	1–7
Sickle cell anemia	0	78–98	0	1–20	1–2
Sickle cell HGB C dis.	0	40–45	40–45	1–10	1–2
Sickle cell thalassemia	0–30	70–95	0	2–30	1–7
Homozygous HGB C dis.	0	0	95–98	1–5	1–2
Thalassemia major	10–90	0	0	10–90	1–5
Hemoglobin C thalassemia	0–35	0	65–85	0–20	1–5

TABLE XX

SICKLE CELL AND HOMOZYGOUS HEMOGLOBIN C DISEASE

	Sickle cell anemia	Sickle cell thalassemia	Sickle cell HGB C disease	Homozygous HGB C disease
Early onset symptoms	++++	+++	++	+
Asthenic habitus	++	+	o	o
Clinical severity	++++	+++	++	+
Hemolytic crises	++++	+++	+	+
Painful crises	+++	++	++++	+
Crises in pregnancy	++	++	+++	o
Enlarged spleen	+	++	+++	++++
Necrosis of bone	++	+	++++	o
Cardiomegaly	+++	++	o	o
Anemia	++++	+++	++	+
Sickling	++++	+++	++	o
Reticulocytosis	++++	+++	+	+
Bilirubinemia	++++	+++	+	+
Microcytosis	o	+	o	o
Target cells	+	+	++	++++
Fetal hemoglobin	++	+++	+	+
Trace of A hemoglobin	o	+	o	o

Sickle cell anemia is by far the most common form of sickle cell disease. It differs from sickle cell hemoglobin C disease in the earlier onset of symptoms and greater degree of hemolytic anemia. Furthermore some patients with sickle cell anemia or sickle cell thalassemia present with a characteristic habitus. This consists of an asthenic appearance with increased arm span, disproportion between the length of the trunk and the legs, and long tapering fingers (95). The patient with sickle cell anemia usually appears younger than the stated age and may show retardation in sexual development, see Figure XXVI. Some children with sickle cell anemia show frontal bossing, prominent upper incisor teeth and a facial appearance similar to children with thalassemia major (Cooley's anemia), see Figure XXV (89). Some children with sickle cell anemia have a greatly distended abdomen due to splenomegaly, Figure XV, or due to a combination of malnutrition and hepatomegaly, Figure XXVIII (160).

The next most common type of sickle cell disease, at least in West Africa, is sickle cell hemoglobin C disease (84). In this condition, the age when first seen in the clinic may be older than in sickle cell anemia, see Figure XXIX. In sickle cell hemoglobin C disease, there may be no symptoms during infancy and only rheumatic pains during early childhood. Symptoms are likely to become aggravated during adolescence.

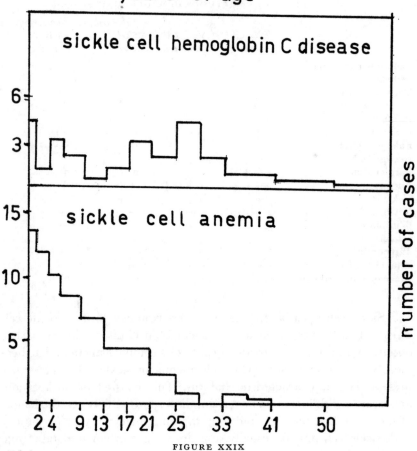

FIGURE XXIX

Pregnancy or delivery may bring on the first serious crisis (43). In males, aseptic necrosis of the head of the femur or hemorrhage into the vitreous portion of the eye may be the first indication of the presence of sickle cell hemoglobin C disease. Splenic infarction is another presenting symptom in this type of sickle cell disease. This is not surprising in view of the fact that splenomegaly may persist through life in sickle cell hemoglobin C disease, even in patients that have never been exposed to malaria (150).

Sickle cell thalassemia is a more unusual variant of sickle cell disease, accounting for less than 10 per cent of those cases found to have mostly S hemoglobin in the electrophoresis. Those few cases of sickle cell thalassemia that have an appreciable amount of A hemoglobin or a large amount of F hemoglobin have a more benign course (168). A rare type of sickle cell disease is sickle cell hemoglobin D disease. Since there are several types of hemoglobin D it is difficult to generalize about the severity of symptons (130). Another rare type of sickle cell disease is sickle cell persistent fetal hemoglobin gene disease. This condition is usually asymptomatic due to the fact that F hemoglobin does not react with S hemoglobin (94).

Homozygous hemoglobin C disease is included in Tables XVIII–XX because the symptons may resemble those of sickle cell disease despite the absence of sickle hemoglobin and sickling (62). Although the life span of the red cells is slightly reduced and target cells are prominent, many individuals remain asymptomatic. Others develop splenomegaly and have both hemolytic and painful episodes. Enlargement of the spleen is characteristic. Just as a fraction of the cases that at first appear to be examples of sickle cell anemia turn out to be cases of sickle cell thalassemia when genetic studies are made, so a fraction of the cases that at first appear to be homozygous hemoglobin C disease turn out to be cases of hemoglobin C thalassemia when genetic studies are made. Hemoglobin C thalassemia is an even milder condition than homozygous hemoglobin C, at least in so far as African cases are concerned (168).

There are both genetic and environmental factors which may modify the course of sickle cell disease. Thus, in sickle cell thalassemia, there are wide variations in the amount of hemoglobin F (1–30 per cent) as well as in the amount of hemoglobin A (0–30 per cent). The amount of A and F hemoglobin in sickle cell thalassemia is probably determined by the genetic character of the beta thalassemia gene that is inherited. This variation is evident in beta thalassemia trait where there may be an elevation of A_2 hemoglobin, F hemoglobin, or either both or neither (168).

In sickle cell anemia there is also wide variation in the percentage of F hemoglobin and this plays a vital role in determining the severity of the disease (65). But, in this disease, the factors responsible for the variation in the level of F hemoglobin are not known. Infants have a higher level than children or adults and on the average females have a higher level than males (17).

An entirely different factor, which may operate in some individuals with sickle cell disease, is the inherited deficiency of the enzyme G-6-P D. Wherever there is a high incidence of sickle hemoglobin, there is a high incidence of this enzyme deficiency as shown in Figures XVI and XX (2) (102). Hence a considerable number of individuals inherit both sickle cell disease and deficiency of G-6-P D. It would seem likely that the inheritance of two red cell abnormalities would result in a clinical picture that was more severe than the inheritance of either abnormality alone. Although the degree of icterus and hyperbilirubinemia is greater in patients with sickle cell anemia and deficiency in G-6-P D, many such patients persue a relatively mild course (87).

A factor which may militate against the well being of the patient with sickle cell disease is splenomegaly (154). This contradicts the statement that "the rare occurrence of splenomegaly in true homozygous sickle cell anaemia is always associated with an unusually bland form of the illness" (49). Even in non-malarial areas, splenomegaly in sickle cell anemia is not rare (22 per cent) and may be associated with a short red cell survival and a low hemoglobin level (144). In malarial areas splenomegaly is more common and hypersplenism may present a problem (84) (89). Even in the absence of splenomegaly, malarial infection has a deleterious effect on the patient with sickle cell disease (58).

Other environmental factors which might play a role in the course of sickle cell disease are the presence or absence of parasitic and bacterial infections other than malaria, nutritional deficiency in iron, folic acid or protein, the general standard of living, and the availability of good medical care.

XI : Sickle Cell Disease in Infancy

SICKLE cell disease in the first two years of life is characterized by several features: the change-over from fetal hemoglobin with its alpha and gamma chains to adult hemoglobin with its alpha and beta chains (161) which results in increasing amounts of S hemoglobin, the development of the hand foot syndrome (166), the advent of hemolytic crises (67) and by frequent severe infections which interfere with the normal growth and development of the infant (148). During the first 3 months of life symptoms due to sickle cell disease are exceedingly rare but during the second 3 months may put in an appearance. Even in the United States, where economic and health standards are high and there is no malaria, 15 per cent of infants, diagnosed as having sickle cell anemia during the first year of life, died within an average follow up period of only six months (120). In Africa, where the conditions are less propitious and malaria is rife, the mortality during the first two years is about 50 per cent (80).

The normal newborn infant has 75–85 per cent of fetal hemoglobin, the premature more and the postmature less. The infant continues to synthesize fetal hemoglobin but the rate of synthesis of adult hemoglobin becomes relatively more rapid so that after 100 days the level of fetal hemoglobin is reduced to approximately 10 per cent. At the age of 15–18 months there is less than one per cent of fetal hemoglobin and this amount remains relatively constant throughout life in a normal individual (161).

In sickle cell trait, the level of fetal hemoglobin follows the same pattern as in infants with a normal hemoglobin pattern, but in sickle cell anemia the level of fetal hemoglobin falls more slowly and may remain indefinitely at a level above normal. However in some patients with sickle cell anemia there is no elevation of the fetal hemoglobin over the normal for the age in question, see Figure XXX (161).

The elevated level of fetal hemoglobin during the first three months of life accounts for the fact that the symptoms of sickle cell disease do not usually occur until some time later. The high level of fetal hemoglobin at birth also makes it difficult to make a laboratory diagnosis of sickle cell disease. To obtain a positive sickling test it may be necessary to combine two techniques, the addition of sodium metabisulfite and

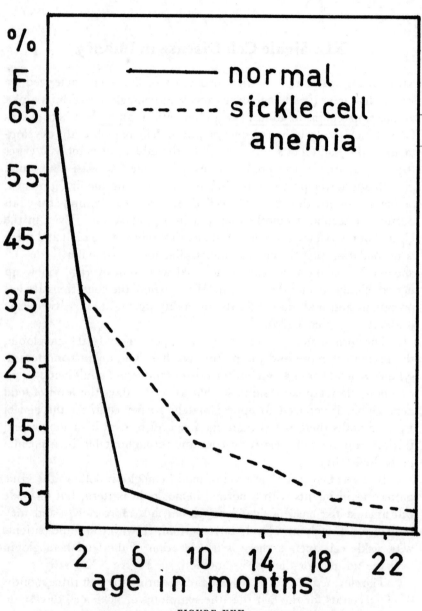

FIGURE XXX
Per centage of fetal hemoglobin during the first two years of life
From Truong *et al.*, 1964.

24 hour incubation of the sealed preparation. Electrophoretic identification is also difficult unless special techniques are used to separate the large amount of fetal hemoglobin from the S hemoglobin which has a similar mobility at alkaline pH. For this purpose it is helpful to use agar gel (72).

Among the signs and symptoms of sickle cell anemia are the presence of hepatomegaly (73%), concurrent infection (70%), failure to thrive (63%), irritability and colic (63%), fever (58%), splenomegaly (50%), abdominal distention (42%), jaundice (36%), dactylitis (37%), pallor (33%), heart murmur (26%), nausea and vomiting (25%) and X-ray evidence of cardiac enlargement (19%). Laboratory studies usually reveal a hemoglobin level of under 9 grams per 100 ml. in the United States (165) and under 7 in Africa (75) except in cases with concomitant G-6-P D defect. Nucleated red blood cells are often present as well as sickled cells (120).

The most characteristic symptom of sickle cell anemia during the first two years of life is swelling of either the hands or feet which may occur in 10–80 per cent of the cases depending upon the peculiarities of the disease as observed in different areas. The clinical features, laboratory findings and x-ray appearance of 20 cases are shown in Table XXI (166).

Fever is an almost constant finding in the early stages of hand foot syndrome, whether related to the thrombotic process or concurrent infection. The swellings are very painful at first, and may persist for many days or weeks. If the feet are involved, the child may refuse to walk. X-ray studies made after symptoms have been present for one or two weeks may show periosteal changes with new bone formation, and in some cases there are destructive lesions of the metacarpals or metatarsals, see Figure XXXI. The age range for this syndrome is quite wide, but the greatest frequency is in children under 3 years of age. The syndrome is more common in sickle cell anemia than sickle cell hemoglobin C disease or sickle cell thalassemia. All of the cases listed in Table XXI had a hemoglobin level over 6 grams and many had 8 or 9 grams per 100 ml. A relatively high hemoglobin level is consistent with the thrombotic nature of the lesion since a very low level would reduce the viscosity of the blood and tend to minimize stagnation and thrombosis. Secondary infection and osteomyelitis of the bones of the hands and feet are rare. Recurrent attacks of the hand foot syndrome are common and often preceded by some form of stress, usually an infection, but sometimes merely a vaccination. The hand foot syndrome is so charac-

TABLE XXI

CLINICAL, LABORATORY AND X-RAY FINDINGS IN HAND FOOT
SYNDROME

Age years	HGB SS	HGB level gm/ 100 ml	WBC 1,000/ cmm	Swelling of hand	foot	Dura- tion days	Subperio- steal new bone	Bone destruc- tion
6/12	+	8·0	19	0	+	21+	+	+
9/12	+	6·1	25	+	+	25	+	+
9/12	+	8·1	55	+	+	21	+	0
10/12	+	8·8	16	0	+	5	0	0
10/12	+	9·1	13	0	+	8	+	0
11/12	+	6·9	21	0	+	4	—	—
11/12	+	7·0	14	+	+	7	0	0
13/12	+	8·0	16	+	+	7	0	0
13/12	+	7·2	23	+	+	28	+	+
15/12	+	9·0	22	+	+	11	+	0
16/12	+	8·2	13	+	+	7	—	—
2	+	7·0	19	+	0	17	+	+
2	+	7·5	—	+	0	17	+	+
2	+	7·1	16	+	+	9	+	0
2 6/12	SC	10·2	14	+	0	14	0	0
2 6/12	+	9·0	8	+	0	—	0	0
4	+	8·0	—	+	+	—	+	0
4 6/12	+	7·8	15	+	+	21	+	0
6	+	8·0	21	0	+	21	0	0
7	+	6·5	14	0	+	4	—	—
AVERAGE		7·9	19	14/20	16/20	14	11/17	5/17

From Watson *et al.*, 1963

teristic of sickle cell anemia that when it occurs in an African child, sickle cell disease should be taken for granted until the diagnosis is disproven.

Although the hand foot syndrome is a disturbing event in the life of the infant with sickle cell disease, it is not associated with any mortality. The serious and fatal complications of sickle cell anemia in infancy are infections and hemolytic crises, see Table XXII. In 64 cases of sickle cell anemia that were diagnosed before one year of age and followed for an average period of six months, there were ten deaths. Eight of the ten had infections and two had crises. The average hemoglobin level in these cases was 5·5 grams compared with 7·9 in the series with hand foot syndrome. Respiratory infection, particularly pneumonia, was the most common cause of death (120). In addition there were two infants that died with septicemia and one each with meningitis and intestinal infection. Apparently the two types of bacteria

TABLE XXII

MORTALITY IN SICKLE CELL ANEMIA IN THE FIRST YEAR

Age at diagnosis months	Number in the group	Number that died	Age at death months	Cause of death	HGB level gm/ 100 ml
1	3	1	2	Pseudomonas sepsis	7·8
2	1	1	3	Pneumonia	4·8
3	4	2	4	Crisis	8·0
				Diarrhoea and acidosis	5·6
4	8	1	11	Pneumonia	2·0
5	6	0	—	—	—
6	6	1	8	Salmonella sepsis	3·6
7	1	0	—	—	—
8	6	1	8	Crisis	3·2
9	10	1	9	Pneumonia, cardiac failure	2·6
10	9	0	—	—	—
11	5	1	11	H. influenza meningitis	6·3
12	5	1	12	Staphylococcal pneumonia	5·9

AVERAGE   (64)   (10)   7·2   5·5
From Porter and Thurman, 1963.

that have a special predilection for individuals with sickle cell hemo-globin are salmonella (118) (121) and pneumococci (132). Pneumococci produce more than a fair share of meningitis cases in infants with sickle cell disease. The reasons for this increased susceptibility to bacterial infections may be chronic anemia, abnormal splenic function, or a tendency for capillary thromboses. The cases listed in Tables XXI–XXIII come from the United States so that an effect from malaria is excluded (67) (120) (166).

Acute hemolytic crises, whether preceded by infection or occurring without evident cause, are another serious and sometimes fatal complication of sickle cell anemia and sickle cell thalassemia during the first two years of life. Ten such cases are analyzed in Table XXIII (67). Here the average hemoglobin level was less than 2·4 grams compared with 5·5 in cases with infection and 7·9 in cases with hand foot syndrome. Not all patients with hemolytic crises show jaundice (67). Fever and convulsions are common. Post mortem examination of seven of the infants listed in Table XXIII showed occasional pulmonary vessel thromboses and capillary engorgement of the cerebral cortex, but more frequently engorgement of the visceral organs. Pooling of blood in the spleen and liver may contribute to the sudden aggravation of the anemia (66).

TABLE XXIII

SUDDEN DEATH IN INFANTS WITH SICKLE CELL ANEMIA

Age years	Pallor	Fever	Convul- sions	Hepato- megaly	Spleno- megaly	Jaundice	HGB level gm/100 ml
8/12	+	+	o	o	o	o	—
1 4/12	+	+	?	+	+	o	<2·5
1 4/12	+	+	+	+	+	+	—
1 5/12	+	o	+	+	+	o	<1·0
1 6/12	+	+	+	o	o	o	<3·0
1 7/12	+	+	o	+	o	o	—
2 5/12	+	o	+	o	+	o	—
4	+	o	o	+	+	+	—
4	+	+	o	o	o	+	—
9	+	o	o	+	+	o	<3·0
AVER- AGE	10/10	6/10	4/10	6/10	6/10	3/10	<2·4

From Jenkins, Scott and Baird, 1960.

In Africa, probably as a result of malarial infection and malnutrition during the weaning period, the mortality of sickle cell anemia during the first two years of life is very high. Some 300 cases were observed in the Congo from 1948 to 1954 and half of them died during the period of observation. The only optimistic comment made by the investigators was that as the children grew older the mortality rate declined (80).

XII : Sickle Cell Disease in Childhood

THE CHILD with sickle cell disease that has survived the first two years of life may have achieved a relatively steady state, adjusting to the physical drawbacks of the disease. Hand foot syndrome and hemolytic crises may become less frequent. On the other hand, abdominal crises occur (159), occasionally aplastic crises (27), hepatic crises (60) or painful vascular occlusive crises (37).

The steady state, see Table XXIV, is marked by anemia, usually

TABLE XXIV

ANALYSIS OF EVENTS IN SICKLE CELL DISEASE

The steady state	Types of crisis	Complications
Anemia	Hemolytic	Osteoporosis
Short RBC life span	Hyperhemolytic (hypersplenism)	Aseptic necrosis
Reticulocytosis		Pathological fracture
Hyperbilirubinemia	Aplastic (reticulocytopenia)	Osteomyelitis
Erythroid hyperplasia	Hand foot syndrome	Fat embolism
Splenomegaly	Bone pain	Skin ulcers
Lymphadenopathy	Joint pain	Gross hematuria
Cardiomegaly	Abdominal pain	Retinal hemorrhage
Hepatomegaly	Hepatic crisis	Retinal detachment
Hepatic dysfunction	Splenic infarct	Vitreous hemorrhage
Folic acid deficiency	Pulmonary infarct	Glaucoma
Hyposthenuria	Bone infarct	Meningismus
Microscopic hematuria	Priapism	Hemiplegia
Epistaxis	Cerebral infarct	Encephalopathy
Local swellings	Generalized sickling	Cor pulmonale
Arthralgia	Combinations of the above	Pericarditis
Delayed growth		Cardiac failure
Delayed maturation		Cirrhosis
Enlarged marrow space		Cholelithiasis
Enlarged diploic space		Thromboses
Slender habitus		Gross infarction
Long tapering fingers		Hemosiderosis
Frontal bossing		

less severe than in the first two years of life. There is a constant reti-culocytosis and slight hyperbilirubinemia with fluctuations at the time of crises. To maintain the level of hemoglobin, the bone marrow becomes hyperplastic and the medullary cavities of the long bones and skull become enlarged (128). In some cases, the increased rate of destruction of red cells leads to the development of hemosiderosis of the spleen (128).

Headache, weakness and fatigue are a consequence of the ever present anemia which often leads to cardiac enlargement and murmurs of various types. Rarely, cor pulmonale or cardiac failure occur as late developments of the same etiology (107). Figure XXXII depicts a case of sickle cell anemia with hepato-splenomegaly and chronic cardiac failure. This patient had cyanosis and clubbing of the fingers and toes, Figure XXXIII. Despite the presence of systolic and diastolic murmurs, the post mortem examination did not reveal any abnormality of the heart other than hypertrophy and dilatation.

In the absence of malaria, or during antimalarial therapy, the spleen gradually gets smaller (57) but the liver remains enlarged. Even during the steady state, liver function tests, and electrophoretic analysis of serum proteins reveal some abnormality indicative of impaired liver function (60). A few patients develop cirrhosis of the liver or cholestatic jaundice (112) and from the United States there have been several reports of gall stones in patients with sickle cell anemia (73).

A sudden deepening of the jaundice and increase in the level of direct acting bilirubin indicates liver damage from the above mentioned causes or due to focal necroses (18). The sinusoids of the liver may be engorged with sickled cells leading to enlargement of the Kupffer cells and fibrin formation. In rare cases there may be massive infarction of the liver. In other cases the bile canaliculi become plugged but high transaminase activity is unusual. Such liver crises may or may not be associated with symptoms of painful crisis. Furthermore this type of reaction is associated with leukocytosis rather than with leukopenia which is characteristic of viral hepatitis (77). In this connection it is worth repeating the observation that icterus is likely to be more frequent and more severe in those cases of sickle cell anemia which are complicated by concomitant inheritance of G-6-P D deficiency (85).

During the steady state, there is reduced ability to concentrate urine (31) so that nocturia and enuresis are not uncommon in children (108). Microscopic haematuria is another characteristic of the disease and is probably the result of papillary necrosis (54) which occurs in sickle cell trait as well as sickle cell disease. Gross hematuria is another complication of the same process (13).

Priapism is seen in adults with sickle cell hemoglobin C disease, rarely in sickle cell trait but in sickle cell anemia it is not so uncommon and may occur at any age over 5 years (79).

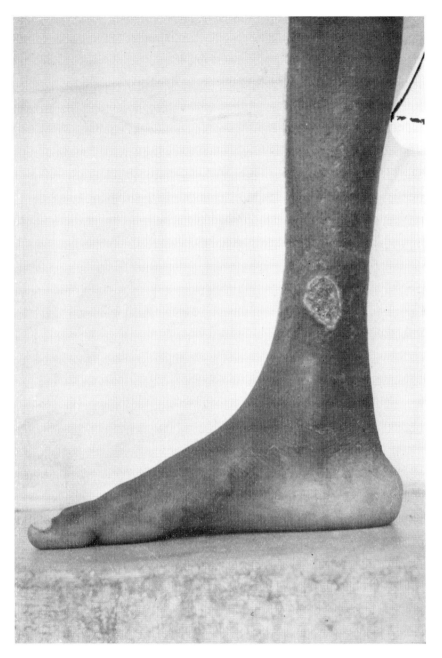

FIGURE XXXVI

Cutaneous ulcer in sickle cell thalassemia

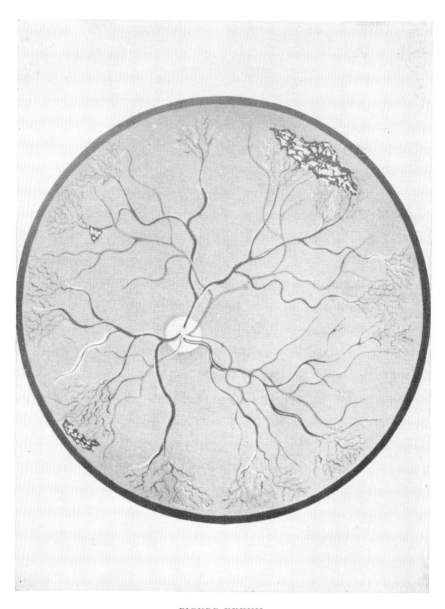

FIGURE XXXVII

Sickle cell retinopathy
From: Lied *et al.*, 1959, modified by Diggs, 1965

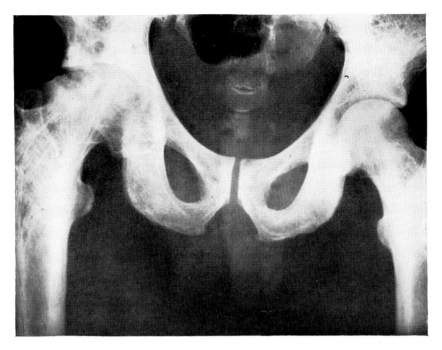

FIGURE XXXVIII

Thinning of the cortex and aseptic necrosis in sickle cell anemia

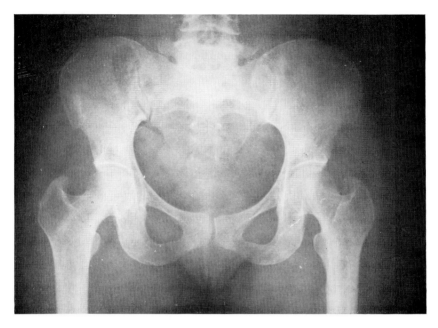

FIGURE XXXIX

Thickening of the cortex in the sickle cell hemoglobin C disease

Nose bleeds and joint pains, localized soft tissue swellings and joint inflammation may occur in the absence of a major crisis. Lymphadenopathy is a characteristic feature of sickle cell disease and may reflect the predisposition to bacterial infections (95).

Some children with sickle cell anemia or sickle cell thalassemia have a slender habitus and almost all appear younger than their actual age. Many children show retardation in sexual development with a late onset of menarche and puberty (71).

The skeletal changes increase during childhood, especially widening of the medullary cavities and osteoporosis. Although the hand foot syndrome is less common during advancing age, some patients develop aseptic necrosis of the head of the femur, see Figure XXXIV. The "bristle brush" appearance of the skull, more characteristic of Cooley's anemia, may develop during childhood, Figure XXXV. Salmonella osteomyelitis may occur in children, in sickle cell hemoglobin C disease as well as in sickle cell anemia (128).

TABLE XXV

RETICULOCYTOPENIC EPISODES IN SICKLE CELL ANEMIA

Age years	Tempera- ture	Infection	PCV %	Reticu- locyte %	Serum bilirubin mg. %	Bone marrow
1 1/12	101·3	Pneumococcal upper resp.	19	0·0	—	Hyperplastic
2 10/12	99·5	Pharyngitis	11	0·4	0·2	Hyperplastic
3	99·4	—	8	0·0	0·8	Hypoplastic
5 6/12	101·5	—	5	0·1	0·1	—
6	98·6	—	6	0·0	1·6	Hypoplastic
8	101·3	Pneumococcal upper resp.	18	1·5	—	—
8	99·5	—	12	0·0	0·3	Hyperplastic
10	104·0	Streptococcal sepsis	16	2·6	1·4	Normal
14	104·7	Pneumococcal pneumonia	12	1·6	2·0	—

From Charney and Miller, 1964.

There are two types of crisis that seem to be more common in childhood than in infancy or in later life, the abdominal crisis and the reticulocytopenic phase or aplastic crisis. The abdominal crisis is marked by fever, muscle splasm, tenderness, nausea, vomiting, leukocytosis and constipation. The last mentioned symptom helps to distinguish the syndrome from acute appendicitis. Even so the condition is difficult to differentiate from other causes of an acute abdomen and surgical intervention is hazardous. It is thought that the symptoms are brought on by an accumulation of sickled cells in the abdominal organs (159).

The aplastic crisis or reticulocytopenic episode is often ushered in by a preceding or concomitant infection, see Table XXV. A fall in the rate of production of red cells leads to a sudden and severe aggravation of the anemia since the high rate of red cell destruction continues unabated (27). This type of crisis is quite different from the anemia complicated by folic acid deficiency which is accompanied by megaloblastic changes in the bone marrow (167).

Central nervous system symptoms are not uncommon during childhood in patients with sickle cell anemia, and may be due to vascular stasis or occlusion in the meninges or cerebral cortex (8). Complications involving the eyes are not as common as in adult life. Ulcers of the skin, especially on the inner aspect of the ankle may occur in older children as well as adults with sickle cell anemia or sickle cell thalassemia (97). Typical vascular occlusive crises with bone or joint pain occur in older children. Splenic and pulmonary infarction are more likely to occur in adults. Hyperhemolytic crises occur in children with hypersplenism. As the child grows older the incidence of crises tends to decline but the number and variety of complications may increase (95) (160).

XIII : Sickle Cell Disease in Adults

ADULTS with sickle cell disease usually have milder symptoms and fewer crises than in childhood except in the case of women during pregnancy. The anemia is likely to be less severe and the hemoglobin level less likely to drop to the low levels that are often encountered during childhood. The individual with sickle cell anemia may enjoy an active career as a teacher or businessman. Some individuals with sickle cell anemia are not so lucky, and there is one case on record of a 27 year old patient living in a large city in the United States who was hospitalized on 97 occasions and required 124 blood transfusions (91). Vascular occlusive crises still occur (37). Furthermore, the adult runs the hazard of complications due to rarifaction of bone, bony infarcts and aseptic necrosis of bone, and vascular lesions affecting the eye. Finally, the adult with sickle cell anemia may succumb to septicemia, respiratory infection, fat embolism, cardiac failure or liver disease, see Table XXVI (26).

TABLE XXVI
CAUSE OF DEATH OF ADULTS WITH SICKLE CELL ANEMIA

Age years	Sex	Cause of death
14	Male	Rheumatic fever and rheumatic heart disease, hepatic necrosis and bone marrow emboli of the lung
15	Male	Massive fat and bone marrow embolization in pulmonary arteries
20	Male	Septicemia with salmonella cholerae suis and cerebral thrombosis.
20	Female	Cirrhosis and hepatic failure.
32	Female	Septicemia with staphylococcus, purulent pericarditis and mitral stenosis
38	Female	Congestive heart failure and pneumonia.
43	Female	Widespread vascular congestion.
46	Female	Abdominal abscess following cholecystectomy, pancreatitis and purulent pericarditis.
48	Male	Multiple myeloma and pneumonia.

From Charache and Richardson, 1964.

The characteristic vascular occlusive crisis of sickle cell disease usually affects the bones or joints and may be felt in the extremities, waist, chest or back. The crisis is due to stasis of blood in the tendons, synovial tissues or bones and the pain often migrates from one place to another during the course of events (37). In a severe crisis, the patient lies grunting and crying with pain, unable to sleep and disinterested in nourishment. The pains may be modified by analgesics but may require parenteral injection of narcotics or tranquilizers (84). The painful crisis is usually accompanied by fever which parallels the severity of the pains which usually last 3–7 days, occasionally longer. There may be swelling of the periarticular soft tissues. The joint pains are aggravated by motion and the bone pains by local pressure. There is often a leukocytosis and the percentage of multipointed sickled cells may increase (37).

Some of the factors which may precipitate painful crises are listed in Table XXVII (78). In Africa the commonest cause is malarial infection. In non-malarial areas bacterial infection is the foremost trigger.

TABLE XXVII

FACTORS LIKELY TO PROVOKE VASCULAR
OCCLUSIVE CRISIS

Malaria
Bacterial infections
Viral infections
Vaccination
Pyrexia
Trauma
Pregnancy
Abortion
Delivery
Anesthesia
Exposure to high altitude
Alcoholic intoxication
Transfusion
Cold weather
Damp weather
Acidosis
Vascular stasis

But viral infection, even vaccination, may initiate a crisis. Trauma, pregnancy, abortion or delivery may initiate a crisis. Low oxygen tension due to anesthesia or airplane flight are additional causative factors. Transfusions, which are useful in the treatment of hemolytic crises may provoke a painful crisis (113). Cold or damp weather seem to be associated with crisis (78). Although patients in the United States seem to do better than those in Africa, the most benign course has been described in individuals living in Jamaica (144). The administration of large doses of ammonium chloride may provoke crisis (10) but acidosis does not seem to play an important role in the genesis of crises (61). At the time of crisis there may be a very low level of folic acid (116) and a very high level of G-6-P D (87), but these may be the result rather than the cause of the crisis. It is important to note that many individuals with sickle cell anemia may undergo the stresses listed in Table XXVII without developing a crisis. Furthermore crises have occurred in the absence of any known predisposing cause (37).

Priapism, or prolonged painful erection, may be considered as a form of crisis or as a complication of sickle cell disease. This condition may arise in children with sickle cell anemia, and in adults with sickle cell disease or sickle cell trait (79). Originally described in the United States, this condition is now known to occur frequently in Africa (79) as well as other tropical countries (144). The duration of priapism may be a matter of days or weeks. Apparently the sickled blood becomes very viscous but does not clot. Recurrent attacks are common.

Another complication of sickle cell anemia that occurs in adults as well as children is cutaneous ulceration on the lower extremities (144) see Figure XXXVI. Peptic ulcer is not unusual in male patients with sickle cell disease (84) (144).

Eye changes are common, and the ophthalmologist may be the first person to make the diagnosis of sickle cell disease. The conjunctivae may show capillary ectasia or corkscrew shaped vessel fragments with proliferation of the endothelial cells. The retina may show small hemorrhages similar to those seen in hypertensive cardiovascular disease, or angioid streaks which are copper coloured irridescent deposits at the periphery of the retina, see Figure XXXVII (90). In some instances these changes result in retinal detachment. Probably the most common ophthalmological accident that occurs in sickle cell disease, especially sickle cell hemoglobin C disease, is vitreous hemorrhage (104). Vision may be partially impaired or totally lost for a period of weeks or months and repeated hemorrhages may cause permanent damage. Rarely the eye lesions result in glaucoma. Temporary loss of vision in sickle cell disease may also be the result of vascular lesions in the central nervous system (8).

Another important system that is very vulnerable in sickle cell disease is the skeletal framework (7). The underlying cause for some of the changes in sickle cell disease is hyperplasia of the bone marrow leading to thinning of the cortex, widened trabecular patterns, deformities and rarely pathological fractures (100). These changes may be seen in the flat and cancellous bones of the calvarium and trunk, as well as the long bones of the extremities. The frontal bone of the orbital roof may be thickened. The diploic space is widened and at first shows a ground glass appearance, later going on to the bristle brush type of picture in a small percentage of cases, see Figure XXXV. Thinning of the cortex of the long bones is characteristic of sickle cell anemia, see Figure XXXVIII, but in sickle cell hemoglobin C disease the cortex of the long bones may become thickened, see Figure XXXIX. The vertebral bodies may become biconcave and the intervertebral discs biconvex. Kyphosis and scoliosis occur, occasionally vertebral collapse. Even the ribs show widened trabecular patterns due to marrow hyperplasia. These changes are quite different from those noted in infants where bossing of the frontal and pariental bones is common and evanescent lesions of the metacarpals and metatarsals occur in connection with the hand foot syndrome (32) (128).

Thrombosis and infarction of the bony tissues supplied by the end arteries may lead to aseptic necrosis. The head of the humerus and even more often the head of the femur are involved. The infarcted portion of bone appears denser on the x-ray, see Figure XXXVIII. The lesion may be bilateral (146).

Another type of skeletal change which occurs in sickle cell anemia is thrombosis and infarction of the shaft of the long bones, see Figure XL. Alternative sources of blood supply insure that the bone survives permitting calcification and new bone formation. The most serious complication of such types of infarction is the production of bone marrow emboli and pulmonary infarction (25). This sequence of events is not uncommon in pregnancy in sickle cell hemoglobin C disease (43).

Infarction of bone in sickle cell disease is sometimes followed by secondary infection resulting in osteomyelitis. In the early stages, the radiological appearance may resemble that of infarction. Osteomyelitis may lead to sequestration and the formation of a draining sinus. The course is chronic with little local or constitutional reaction (23). There may be multiple foci at the same time or one after the other. The micro-organism usually involved is either a salmonella or staphylococcus (118).

XIV : Sickle Cell Disease and Pregnancy

EXTENSIVE studies have shown that the only abnormality characteristic of pregnancy in women with sickle cell trait is an increased tendency to develop bacteruria and pyelonephritis (170). These renal complications are twice as common in pregnant women with sickle cell trait as in pregnant women with a normal hemoglobin pattern, and may be associated with the fact that individuals with sickle cell trait show hyposthenuria, microscopic hematuria and papillary necrosis (31).

On the other hand, the hazards of pregnancy in sickle cell disease are great. The risks attendant upon pregnancy in sickle cell anemia (6) and sickle cell thalassemia (39) are quite different from the risks of pregnancy in sickle cell hemoglobin C disease (43). Furthermore, the course of pregnancy in sickle cell disease depends on whether the expectant mother is given adequate prenatal care or admitted as an emergency and allowed to deliver before a diagnosis of sickle cell disease has been made (43).

Retardation of growth and development is a characteristic feature of sickle cell anemia and sickle cell thalassemia. Sexual as well as physical development is retarded so that it is not surprising that there is a delay in the onset of menstruation (71), see Table XXVIII. There is also a lower fertility rate which is reflected in the higher average age at the time of the first pregnancy as well as a smaller number of preg-

TABLE XXVIII

SICKLE CELL ANEMIA AND PREGNANCY

	Control group	Sickle cell anemia group
Number delivered in the hospital	91	16
Age range, years	14–40	14–40
Mean age at menarche, years	12·2	13·9
Mean age at first pregnancy	19·9	23·9
Mean number of pregnancies	3·5	2·0
Total number of pregnancies	317	33
Abnormal deliveries, per cent	17	39
Abortions		7
Prematures		5
Still births		1

From Jimenez *et al.*, 1966

nancies. Pregnancy in sickle cell anemia often ends in abortion and there is a higher than usual number of premature and still-births (71). Hospitalization is often necessary during the third trimester because of the frequent development of joint pains as well as the risk of pre-eclampsia (6). Painful crises in sickle cell anemia during pregnancy seem to carry a high risk of pulmonary embolism, whether due to sickled cells or bone marrow fragments (137).

Another hazard of pregnancy in sickle cell anemia is the development of folic acid deficiency and severe anemia (167). Apparently there is an increased need for folic acid during pregnancy and hemolytic anemias so that the combination of pregnancy and sickle cell anemia often leads to lower than normal serum levels of folic acid. However, the administration of folic acid does not always improve the anemia even when the serum level of folic acid is restored to normal (116). On the other hand, in areas where folic acid deficiency is not uncommon, the administration of folic acid to women with sickle cell disease during pregnancy has a beneficial effect on the anemia (167).

It has been said that the risk of pregnancy in sickle cell anemia is less than the risk in sickle cell hemoglobin C disease (33). This may be due to the fact that the patient with sickle cell anemia is so diagnosed before delivery while a certain number of pregnant women with sickle cell hemoglobin C disease are delivered before the existence of sickle cell disease is appreciated. The pregnant woman with sickle cell anemia or sickle cell thalassemia runs the risk of painful crises, aggravation of anemia, development of folic acid deficiency, pulmonary embolism, pre-eclampsia, thrombophlebitis and cardiac failure, see Table XXIX. It has been suggested that in addition to malaria prophylaxis and the

TABLE XXIX

COMPLICATIONS OF SICKLE CELL ANEMIA
DURING PREGNANCY

Number of cases reported	28
Joint pains	21
Pre-eclampsia	5
Abdominal crises	3
Pulmonary embolism	3
Folic acid deficiency	3
Thrombophlebitis	2
Hematuria	1
Cardiac failure	1
Cerebral symptoms	1
Breast abscess	1
Death	1

administration of folic acid, the early delivery by caesarean section is less dangerous than waiting for spontaneous full term delivery (6).

The situation in sickle cell hemoglobin C disease is quite different. Fertility may be normal and abortions are not common. In a series of 147 booked cases, Table XXX, the average number of pregnancies was

TABLE XXX

COMPLICATIONS OF SICKLE CELL HEMOGLOBIN C DISEASE IN PREGNANCY AMONG CASES RECEIVING PRENATAL CARE

Number of cases	147
Previous still-birth	3
Previous caesarean section	9
Average number of pregnancies	2·6
Average weeks gestation when first seen	28
Average Hgb. level when seen (gm/100 ml)	9·1
Palpable spleen	90
Enlarged liver	69
Number of patients having bone pain crises	72
Number having such crises at delivery	33
Number having acute sequestration crises	3
Total number of bone pain crises	93
Number with megaloblastic erythropoesis	24
Number with pseudo-pre-eclampsia	9
Caesarean section	11
Forceps delivery	5
Death before delivery	2
Death after delivery	6
Total number of deaths	8

From Fullerton *et al.*, 1965.

2·6 and there were some women who had more than six (43). Whereas the birth weight of infants from mothers with sickle cell anemia is far below normal, the average birth weight of infants of mothers with sickle cell hemoglobin C disease is only slightly less than normal. On the other hand, the risk of pregnancy to the mother with sickle cell hemoglobin C disease is considerable. Apparently, the chief hazards are severe anemia, bone marrow embolism and pulmonary infarction (25), the over all mortality being as high as 10 per cent in some series. In other series, Table XXXI, the mortality is much smaller (43).

The cases in the first series of Table XXXI were given antimalarial therapy and ferrous sulfate as well as folic acid when erythropoesis was megaloblastic and blood transfusions when the hemoglobin level fell below 8 gm. per 100 ml. In the second series folic acid was

TABLE XXXI

ANALYSIS OF CAUSE OF DEATH IN 190 CASES OF
PREGNANCY IN SICKLE CELL HEMOGLOBIN C DISEASE

Complication	Booked cases			Emergency cases			Grand total
	First series	Next series	Total	First series	Next series	Total	
Number of cases	64	83	147	21	22	43	190
Megaloblastic anemia	2	0	2	2	3	5	7
Bone marrow or fat embolism	2	1	3	2	0	2	5
Acute sequestration	1	0	1	0	0	0	1
Puerperal sepsis	0	0	0	1	0	1	1
Hepatitis	1	0	1	0	0	0	1
Eclampsia	0	1	1	0	0	0	1
Homologous serum jaundice	0	0	0	1	0	0	1
Total deaths	6	2	8	6	3	9	17
Mortality in per cent	9·4	2·4	5·4	29	14	21	9

From Fullerton *et al.*, 1965.

given whether erythropoesis was megaloblastic or not and blood transfusions were withheld until the hemoglobin fell below 6 gm. Furthermore exchange transfusions were given when the hemoglobin level was below 4 gm. Heparin was given to all patients having painful crises during labour or the first 4 days of the puerperium. In these cases it was necessary to administer protamine sulphate before caesarean section when this was indicated. Despite these precautions there was still some risk associated with pregnancy in sickle cell hemoglobin C disease (43).

XV : Sickle Cell Disease and Surgery

THE SURGICAL aspects of sickle cell disease include the differential diagnosis between surgical conditions and events in the course of sickle cell disease that produce similar signs and symptoms, the occurrence of surgical complications due to sickle cell disease, the hazards of anesthesia and operation in sickle cell disease and the use of splenectomy in an attempt to ameliorate the symptoms of sickle cell disease, see Table XXXII.

TABLE XXXII

SURGICAL ASPECTS OF SICKLE CELL DISEASE

I   MANIFESTATIONS RESEMBLING SURGICAL CONDITIONS

    a. abdominal crises : acute abdomen
    b. splenic infarct   : splenic rupture
    c. dactylitis   : osteomyelitis
    d. synoveal infarct : pyo-arthritis
    e. hematuria   : hypernephroma
    f. icterus   : biliary obstruction
    g. osteoporosis   : osteomalacia
    h. aseptic necrosis : Perthe's disease
    i. breast infarct   : breast abscess

II   SURGICAL COMPLICATIONS

    a. epistaxis
    b. chronic ulcer of the skin
    c. aseptic necrosis of head of humerus or femur
    d. osteomyelitis
    e. pathological fracture or vertebral collapse
    f. gall stones
    g. obstetrical complications
    h. priapism
    i. retinal detachment
    j. splenic rupture or infection or infarct

III   SURGICAL PROCEDURES WITH INCREASED HAZARD

    a. stasis (due to application of tourniquet)
    b. anoxia (due to anesthesia)
    c. hypothermia (due to anesthesia)
    d. metabolic acidosis (due to anesthesia)
    e. crises following transfusion reaction
    f. thrombophlebitis due to inactivity or immobilization

IV   SURGICAL PROCEDURES USED IN THE TREATMENT

    a. splenectomy for hypersplenism in sickle cell anemia
    b. splenectomy for enlarged spleen in sickle cell hemoglobin C disease

In young children it is difficult to distinguish between an abdominal crisis brought on by sickling and an acute abdomen brought on by appendicitis or some other abdominal catastrophe. The abdominal crisis is marked by vomiting, fever, leukocytosis, pain, tenderness and local rigidity. The frequent occurrence of constipation and of slight jaundice suggests a sickling crisis. The x-ray may show fluid levels in the intestine. The child is likely to show splenomegaly and hepatomegaly. Laparotomy in such cases is useless and dangerous, revealing only slight, blood stained peritoneal effusion. The chief lesion is multiple mesenteric capillary occlusions (159).

In the adult, abdominal crises are unusual except in pregnancy, but splenic infarction may occur giving signs and symptoms similar to splenic rupture. If the condition arises soon after an airplane flight, splenic infarction is easy to diagnose (134). But in spontaneous cases there may be confusion with other abdominal conditions which can produce peritoneal irritation and surgical shock (109). Actual rupture of the spleen or abscess formation in the infarcted area are rare complications that do call for surgical intervention (118).

Dactylitis, or hand foot syndrome, may resemble tuberculous involvement or osteomyelitis of the small bones of the hand or foot (166). In fact a small number of children with hand foot syndrome go on to develop osteomyelitis. In the early stages the x-ray does not help with the diagnosis (128). When the swellings last for several weeks x-ray changes become apparent. The administration of antibiotics does no harm when the condition is due to sickling alone, but chloramphenicol should not be given unless there is good evidence of infection. Synoveal infarcts may produce warm tender joints that resemble arthritis of pyogenic origin (109).

Gross hematuria occurs in sickle cell trait, and sickle cell disease. The pyelogram may show a filling defect (86) thus complicating the diagnosis. In tropical areas microscopic hematuria due to bilharzia is difficult to distinguish from hematuria due to sickling.

Intense jaundice in sickle cell disease may have some of the characteristics of obstructive jaundice (112). But clay coloured stools are not found in hepatitis due to sickle cell disease. Other cases of liver crisis (77) may be mistaken for amebic hepatitis or amebic abscess of the liver.

Aseptic necrosis of the head of the femur can be distinguished from Perthe's disease because the outer third of the head is usually spared and the metaphysis is not affected (146). Aseptic necrosis in sickle cell disease may be bilateral, see Figure XXXIV. The condition may heal spontaneously and gradually if weight bearing is avoided. However, in adults, it may be necessary to resort to orthopedic procedures such as osteotomy, arthrodesis or the use of a prosthesis (48).

Soft tissue infarcts of muscle or glandular tissue may be confused with abscess formation but are usually accompanied by other signs and symptoms of sickle cell disease if not an acute crisis.

Among the surgical complications of sickle cell disease, the most common is ulceration of the skin affecting the lower extremity, especially in older children and young adults. In some cases the ulcer heals with simple treatment. However, some ulcers persist for years. Bed rest and the use of elastic bandages have helped in some cases. In others repeated transfusions have led to healing (28). Skin grafting of various types has been tried and although not always successful this method may reduce the period of hospitalization (51).

TABLE XXXIII

CASES OF OSTEOMYELITIS IN ELIZABETHVILLE

	Sickle cell anemia	other children
Number of cases	16	22
Salmonella	13	0
Staphylococci	2	21
Streptococci	0	1
Not determined	1	0
Solitary lesions	5	19
Multiple lesions	11	3
Male children	4	14
Female children	12	8
0–6 months of age	0	2
½–3 years of age	2	2
3–6 years of age	12	4
6–10 years of age	2	9
Over 10 years old	0	5
Fatal cases	0	1

From Pieters et Lambotte, 1965.

Osteomyelitis is much more common in individuals with sickle cell disease than in persons with a normal hemoglobin pattern. Multiple lesions and salmonella infection are characteristic features of osteomyelitis in sickle cell disease (118), see Table XXXIII.

Vertebral collapse and pathological fractures may occur in sickle cell disease and require surgical treatment (109). Epistaxis is a common event in sickle cell anemia in children but does not present any therapeutic problem. On the other hand, priapism may persist despite medical and surgical measures (79) though sequelae are less common when medical treatment is employed. Gallstones have been found in cases of sickle cell anemia but most of the reports have emanated from the United States as this complication is rare in Africa (68).

The hazards of surgery in sickle cell disease may be due to stasis, hypothermia, anoxia or acidosis. Stasis may be caused by tight bandaging, the application of a cast, or the use of a tourniquet. These measures must be used with caution in patients with sickle cell disease lest a crisis be precipitated (22).

Hypothermia produces circulatory stasis, and although it may decrease the rate of oxygen utilization it is dangerous in sickle cell disease. Immersion of the hand in ice water will elicit the hand foot syndrome (99). Even individuals with sickle cell trait may develop circulatory damage if exposed to hypothermia (164).

Ether anesthesia often entails a degree of anoxia due to the reduction in respiratory volume. The tendency to anoxia is greater when nitrous oxide is used. Fatalities have been reported following tonsillcetomy (133) or removal of a ganglion at the wrist (46). The need for maintaining full oxygenation during anesthesia is especially important in patients with sickle cell disease (30).

An approach to the management of the patient with sickle cell disease when elective surgery is contemplated is to replace the sickle hemoglobin with normal hemoglobin by repeated transfusions (38). When the hemoglobin level reaches normal the patient stops producing red cells. However, transfusions in sickle cell disease are not without hazard. It is possible to transmit homologous serum jaundice or to elicit a crisis and there is the danger of producing hemosiderosis.

Finally, the surgeon is sometimes requested to perform a splenectomy to ameliorate the course of a patient with sickle cell disease. In hypersplenism, even the normal red cells given by transfusion are rapidly destroyed and hemolytic crises are difficult to control (89). The half life of the patient's red cells is incredibly short (40). Thus, in sickle cell anemia (40) and sickle cell thalassemia (89), splenectomy may be a life saving procedure. On the other hand, it is considered unwise to carry out a splenectomy when the spleen is functioning normally. In sickle cell anemia there is a gradual reduction in the size of the spleen due to repeated infarction so that "autosplenectomy" may be anticipated. But in sickle cell hemoglobin C disease it may be advisable to remove a greatly enlarged spleen to ameliorate symptoms and prevent subsequent infarction or rupture. Following splenectomy it is necessary to guard against malaria infection and there may be increased susceptibility to bacterial and viral disease (155).

XVI : Carbohydrate Metabolism of the Red Cell

THE RED cells are peculiarly adapted for the transport of oxygen, using little for their own metabolism and having special mechanisms to protect against oxidative processes. Utilization of oxygen by stagnant blood is due to the presence of leukocytes, platelets and reticulocytes (89A). Furthermore, the red cell contains chiefly potassium ions sur-

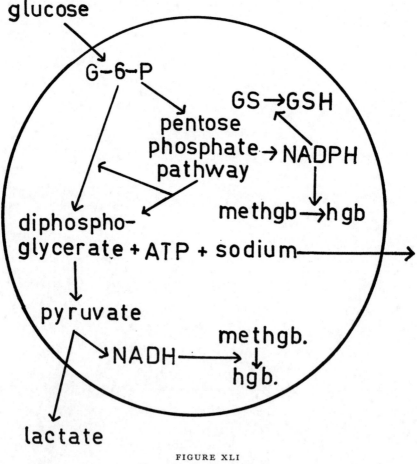

FIGURE XLI
Normal red cell metabolism

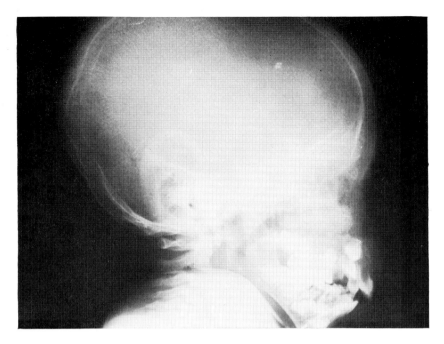

FIGURE XXXV

Enlargement of diploic space and hair on end appearance in sickle cell anemia

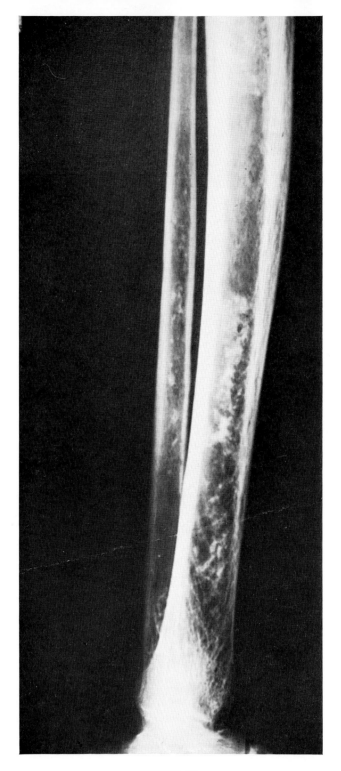

FIGURE XL

Infarct of bone in sickle cell disease

rounded by a sea of sodium ions. To maintain this state of affairs, the red cell needs a constant supply of oxygen.

The energy for the metabolism of the red cell is derived from glucose, most of which is converted to lactate, see Figure XLI. Elsewhere in the body, the lactate is further oxidized or converted back to glucose. Glucose in the red cell reaches the lactic acid stage through the Emden-Meyerhof pathway, anaerobic, generating ATP (adenosine triphosphate) and NADH or DPNH (reduced adenine dinucleotide) or (diphosphopyridine nucleotide). The ATP is required for several enzyme reactions including those involved in the pump which keeps sodium ions out of the red cell. The NADH is required for other enzyme systems such as NADH dependent methemoglobin reductase (98).

However, more than 10 per cent of the glucose consumed by the red cell passes through the pentose phosphate pathway yielding 25 per cent of the energy (14).

Oxidation of glucose through the pentose phosphate pathway yields NADPH or TPNH (reduced nicotinamide adenine dinucleotide phosphate) or (reduced triphosphopyridine nucleotide). The NADPH is also required for enzyme reactions, in particular, the transformation of glutathione to reduced glutathione and the reduction of methemoglobin to hemoglobin by the NADPH dependent methemoglobin reductase. These reactions protect the red cell against the action of oxidant drugs. The NADPH is also required for enzyme reactions involved in maintenance of the integrity of the lipid membrane that surrounds the red cell (24).

Figure XLII gives a more detailed summary of the Emden-Meyerhof pathway showing the stage where some of the glucose-6-phosphate is diverted to the pentose phosphate pathway. Three molecules of glucose or 18 carbon atoms yield three of ribulose and three of carbon dioxide. The three molecules of ribulose form one molecule of glyceraldehyde and two of fructose, thus accounting for all 18 of the carbon atoms (14).

Reduced glutathione forms the main buffer system against oxidation and this explains why the red cell has such a high content of glutathione, most of which is reduced. The level approximates that of glucose, 100 mg. per 100 ml. of red cells. Patients with a congenital deficiency of glutathione or its reductase manifest the same type of hemolytic anemia as individuals with G-6-P D deficiency. Reduced glutathione protects sulfhydryl groups and hemoglobin against oxida-

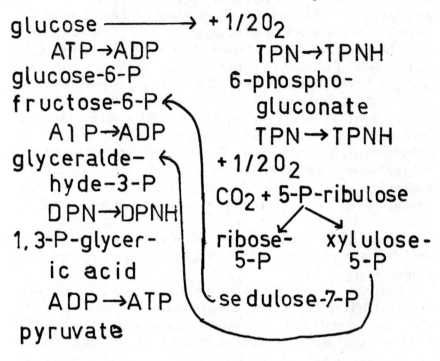

FIGURE XLII
Glucose metabolism

tion, neutralizes hydrogen peroxide and maintains the integrity of the cell wall (15).

Congenital abnormalities of the enzymes of the Emden-Meyerhof cycle, deficiency of pyruvate kinase, 2-3-diphosphoglyceromutase, or triose phosphate isomerase, may produce a congenital hemolytic anemia (24).

Abnormalities in the enzymes of the pentose phosphate pathway, deficiency of glucose-6-phosphate dehydrogenase, 6-phosphogluconate dehydrogenase, glutathione reductase or lack of glutathione may produce a form of non-spherocytic hemolytic anemia and render the red cells susceptible to hemolysis after the administration of oxidant drugs (15). Under these circumstances reduced glutathione is converted to glutathione and hemoglobin to methemoglobin. The methemoglobin agglomerates and is further oxidized to form an insoluble polymer which appears as Heinz bodies in red cells when they are stained with supravital dyes such as crystal violet (42). Analogous inclusion bodies are formed from the polymerization of the relatively unstable hemoglobin H and hemoglobin M (156).

Deficiency of methemoglobin reductase may cause methemoglobinemia but there is neither hemolysis nor anemia (171).

All of the congential defects in red cell metabolism that have been mentioned are relatively rare, especially in Africans, except for deficiency of the enzyme G-6-P D or glucose-6-phosphate dehydrogenase. Although the extreme form of this deficiency may lead to congenital non-spherocytic anemia, the form that occurs with great frequency in Africans only leads to anemia as a complication of certain diseases and the administration of certain drugs (169).

XVII : Glucose-6-Phosphate Dehydrogenase Variants

THE MOST important enzyme in the pentose phosphate pathway is glucose-6-phosphate dehydrogenase or G-6-P D. In technical terms, the amount of this enzyme is the rate limiting factor for the quantity of glucose which can be oxidized by the pentose phosphate pathway (24).

Peculiarly enough, there are several different variants of the enzyme G-6-P D, and those variants that exhibit reduced activity are found frequently in those parts of the world where falciparum malaria has been prevalent, so that the distribution of individuals with reduced enzyme activity coincides with the distribution of abnormal hemoglobins (92), see Figure XVI. However, the exact chemical constitution of G-6-P D has not been determined, and its variants are characterized by their enzymatic potency, their electrophoretic mobility and other physico-chemical measurements (127).

The normal and most universally distributed type is called B. In northern Europe and in the original inhabitants of the "New World" it is extremely unusual to find any other variants of G-6-P D. However, in Africa, there is a high incidence of A and A— variants. In fact, in many parts of Africa south of the Sahara some 20 per cent of the G-6-P D genes are A and 20 per cent A—, leaving only 60 per cent of the genes as the normal type B, see Table XXXIV (127). This Table

TABLE XXXIV
COMMON G–6–P D VARIANTS

Where found	Apparent frequency in Africa	Name of variant	Activity per cent of B	Electrophoretic mobility per cent of B
Universal	60%	B	100	100
Africans	20%	A	88	110
Africans	20%	A—	8–20	110
Greece	0	Greek	12–45	100
South China	0	Canton	4–15	105
Europe and Asia	0	Mediterranean	0–7	100

includes the common Mediterranean variant which bears the name of the geographical region where it is most frequently encountered. This variant has the same electrophoretic properties as B, but a greatly reduced enzyme activity. The "normal" African variant A has about 90 per cent of the activity of B while A— has only about 10 per cent of the activity of B. Both A and A— have a more rapid rate of migration in an electric field, and can be distinguished from B by electrophoresis. In Greece and in parts of China, there are G-6-P D variants with severely reduced activity. There are rare and isolated instances of G-6-P D variants with either greater than normal, normal, or almost no enzymatic activity (127).

As in the case of inheritance of abnormal hemoglobins, the gene for G-6-P D exerts partial dominance. But in contrast with the inheritance of abnormal hemoglobins which is determined by genes on the ordinary chromosomes or autosomes, the gene for G-6-P D is located on the female chromosome. As a result of this sex linked inheritance, the male has only one gene and the female has two for the inheritance of G-6-P D. Thus in the African female, one may find AA, AB or BB patterns with practically normal activity, AA— and BA— with slightly reduced activity, and A—A— with markedly reduced activity. But in the African male, one can find only A and B with practically normal activity and A— with markedly reduced activity, see Table XXXV.

TABLE XXXV

G-6-P D PATTERNS IN AFRICANS

	Electrophoretic patterns					
Male	B	A				A—
Female	BB	AB	AA	BA—	AA—	A—A—
Activity		Normal +			Variable +—	Defect —

The sex linked character of the inheritance of G-6-P D leads to two interesting phenomenon. The male child inherits his G-6-P D gene from the mother, while the female child inherits her G-6-P D genes from both the father and mother. To simplify matters, one may designate A and B variants as + and A— as —. The possible types of inheritance in the African are shown in Table XXXVI. Inheritance of two + genes gives a normal homozygous female, while one + gene gives a normal hemizygous male. Similarly inheritance of two — genes gives an abnormal homozygous female while one — gene gives

TABLE XXXVI

INHERITANCE OF G-6-P D IN AFRICANS

A and B designated by +
A—   designated by —

Assuming a 20 per cent incidence of A—

51·2% of matings		12·8% of matings	
mother	father	mother	father
++	+	++	—
girls	boys	girls	boys
++ ++	+ +	+— +—	+ +

25·6% of matings		6·4% of matings	
mother	father	mother	father
+—	+	+—	—
girls	boys	girls	boys
++ +—	+ —	+— ——	+ —

3·2% of matings		0·8% of matings	
mother	father	mother	father
——	+	——	—
girls	boys	girls	boys
+— +—	— —	—— ——	— —

an abnormal hemizygous male. Only the female has the possibility of heterozygous inheritance of G-6-P D.

The heterozygous female may show a preponderance of red cells with normal enzyme activity or a preponderance of red cells with reduced enzyme activity. This condition is due to the tendency for one of the genes on the female chromosome to predominate. Furthermore, in the heterozygous female, some of the red cells may have a low enzyme activity while other red cells may have a normal enzyme activity. Thus, the red cells of the heterozygous female may have a mosaic pattern with different enzyme activity in different cells (14).

In individuals with G-6-P D variants that show marked deficiency in G-6-P D, tissues other than the red cell may be affected. However, most of the disturbances which occur in such individuals are due to the peculiar metabolism of the red cells. Among the clinical disturbances are jaundice and hemolysis (15).

Infants born with a deficiency in the enzyme G-6-P D may develop neonatal jaundice. Later in life there may be hemolysis, with or without jaundice, as the result of disease, drug administration or the ingestion of certain foods such as the fava bean (76). The jaundice in viral hepatitis is likely to be more marked in those individuals who show a deficiency in G-6-P D (29).

Hemolysis associated with the ingestion of fava beans has never been reported in Africans despite the large number that have the enzyme deficiency. This may be due to the fact that Africans do not eat fava beans, or due to the fact that the enzyme deficiency in Africans is less severe than in individuals of Mediterranean descent (15). The various clinical conditions, and the enzyme variants with which they are associated are listed in Table XXXVII.

TABLE XXXVII

CLINICAL EFFECTS OF G-6-P D VARIANTS

Name of variant	Viral hepatitis affected	Neonatal jaundice	Drug hemolysis	Favism	Congenital nonspherocytic anemia
B	o	o	o	o	o
A	o	o	o	o	o
A—	+	+	+	o	o
Greek	+	+	+	o	o
Canton	+	+	+	o	+
Mediterranean	+	+	+	+	o

XVIII : Diagnosis and Distribution of G-6-P D Deficiency

HEMOLYSIS in American Negroes following the administration of pamaquine, otherwise known as plasmochin, was noted before the mechanism of action was understood. This phenomenon has been carefully studied with a similar but less toxic antimalarial, primaquine. Deficiency of the enzyme G-6-P D is now often referred to as primaquine-type sensitivity despite the fact that the hemolytic reaction may be produced by any of the drugs listed in Table XXXVIII. A clinical diagnosis of G-6-P D deficiency may be entertained when a hemolytic

TABLE XXXVIII

DRUG HEMOLYSIS IN THE AFRICAN TYPE OF G-6-P D DEFICIENCY

Chemical type	Drug	Daily dose	Degree of hemolysis
8-amino-quinoline	pamaquine	30 mg.	very severe
	primaquine	30 mg.	severe
	pentaquine	30 mg.	severe
	quinocide	30 mg.	severe
hydrazine	phenylhydrazine	90 mg.	severe
sulfonamides	sulfanilamide	4 gm.	moderate
	sulfacetamide	4 gm.	moderate
	sulfapyridine	4 gm.	severe
	sulfamethoxypyridazine	2 gm.	moderate
	salicylazosulfapyridine	6 gm.	severe
	sulfisoxazole	8 gm.	moderate
sulfones	thiazolsulfone	3 gm.	moderate
	sulfoxone	300 mg.	slight
	dapsone	200 mg.	moderate
nitrofuranes	nitrofurazone	1·5 gm.	slight
	nitrofurantoin	0·5 gm.	moderate
	furazolidone	0·5 gm.	moderate
	furaltadone	1·0 gm.	moderate
anilines	acetanilide	4 gm.	moderate
	acetophenetidin	4 gm.	moderate
	aminopyrine	2 gm.	slight
4-amino-quinoline	chloroquine	300 mg.	slight
	quinacrine	100 mg.	slight
	methylene blue	400 mg.	slight
phenols	acetylsalicylic acid	12 gm.	slight
napthaquinones	menadione*	2·5 mg.	slight

* newborn infants

reaction occurs in an African following the administration of one of these drugs, especially when the hemolytic reaction starts 2 or 3 days after the drug is started and when the hemolytic reaction is self limited (3).

Neonatal jaundice, appearing a few days after the birth of an African child should also evoke suspicion of G-6-P D deficiency. The diagnosis can be strengthened by eliminating ABO and Rh incompatibility by the appropriate laboratory tests. The figures given in Table XXXIX indicate that in Ghana, the occurence of severe jaun-

TABLE XXXIX

ROLE OF G-6-P D DEFICIENCY AND Rh AND ABO
INCOMPATIBILITY IN NEONATAL JAUNDICE

Group	Number	G-6-P D defect %	ABO incom- patibility %	Rh incom- patibility %
Normals	153	13·6	16·3	5·1
Jaundiced	105	39·0	22·9	2·9
Bilirubin over 25 mg.%	33	63·6	0·0	3·0
Bilirubin over 25 mg.% and fatal	10	100·0	0·0	10·0*

* One patient with both G-6-P D defect and Rh incompatibility.

dice in the neonatal period is usually associated with G-6-P D defect (45). On the other hand, it should be noted that the presence of G-6-P D defect does not always lead to neonatal jaundice. Furthermore, infants of African ancestry born in the United States have been carefully observed for neonatal jaundice in association with G-6-P D defect and this has not occurred except in premature infants (109). Apparently additional factors are involved in determining whether jaundice occurs (45).

A clinical diagnosis of G-6-P D defect may be entertained when an individual with viral hepatitis, sickle cell disease, or almost any other type of infection (169) develops jaundice out of all proportion to the other signs and symptoms of the disease. Proof of the diagnosis of G-6-P D defect depends upon laboratory tests of the patient's blood. But during the acute hemolytic phase the presence of defect may be masked and it may be necessary to take a sample during convalescence (139) or from the parents of the patient.

There are many different laboratory tests for G-6-P D activity and these have been listed in the order of their development in Table XL.

TABLE XL

METHODS FOR THE DETECTION OF G-6-P D DEFICIENCY

Type of test	Author	Date
Heinz body formation on incubation with acetylphenylhydrazine	Beutler	1955
Reduction in level of reduced glutathione on incubation	Beutler	1957
Spectrophotometric determination of TPNH formation	Zinkham	1958
Reduction of brilliant cresyl blue	Motulsky	1961
Reduction of dimethylthiazolydiphenyltetrazolium	Fairbanks	1962
Reduction of methemoglobin formed by nitrite	Brewer	1960–2
Ascorbic acid cyanide test	Rabjtzis	1964
Methylene blue reduction test	Oski	1965
Reduction of methemoglobin in individual cells	Tonz	1965
Spot test of fluorescence due to production of TPNH	Beutler	1966

The microscopic observation of Heinz bodies in blood incubated with acetylphenylhydrazine was the first test to be employed (157). However, it is tedious to perform and non-specific so that other methods are now used. A more specific but equally complicated method is to measure the level of reduced glutathione before and after incubation of whole blood. A sharp drop in the level of reduced glutathione is indicative of enzyme deficiency (15).

The most accurate method of estimating G-6-P D activity is the quantitative spectrophotometric assay based on the rate of formation of TPNH (NADPH) due to the oxidation of G-6-P and its intermediate product 6-phosphogluconate. Two assays must be carried out, one using G-6-P as the substrate, the other with 6-phosphogluconate (24).

A simpler test for G-6-P D deficiency is the so-called methemoglobin reduction test. In this method blood is taken with an anticoagulant other than oxalate since oxalate ions inhibit the enzyme (21). Two reagents are added, one containing methylene blue which acts as a catalyst for G-6-P D, and the other containing sodium nitrite which converts hemoglobin to methemoglobin. The methemoglobin is reduced to hemoglobin by a diaphorase that requires the TPNH generated by the action of G-6-P D. The method is sensitive enough to detect partial or heterozygous deficiency (20). In cases of moderate hemolytic anemia it may reveal the presence of congenital deficiency of the enzyme despite the higher levels caused by the presence of younger red cells (87). To verify the diagnosis of G-6-P D deficiency it is useful to test the mother of male children and both parents of female children.

An interesting modification of the methemoglobin reduction test is its application to blood smears where it reveals the variation in activity of G-6-P D which is characteristic of female heterozygotes (44).

If the incidence of G-6-P D defect in the male population is Q per cent, then the incidence of normals in the male population is $100-Q$ per cent. In the same population the incidence of homozygous G-6-P D defect in females would be Q^2 per cent. The incidence of heterozygous or partial defect in females would then be $2Q(100-Q)$ per cent, and the incidence of normal females $(100-Q)^2$ per cent. The total of homozygous and heterozygous cases of G-6-P D defect in the female would be $2Q - Q^2$ per cent or a little less than double the rate of hemizygous defect in males (24).

Since most of the screening tests for G-6-P D defect miss about half of the heterozygous cases, the figure obtained for the incidence is almost the same for males, females or the total population. But the figure that is obtained with males alone is more reliable (127).

TABLE XLI

INCIDENCE OF G-6-P D VARIANTS AND G-6-P D DEFICIENCY IN AFRICA

Country	Sector	B(%)	A(%)	A−(%)
Algeria				0–12
Angola				17–27
Bechuanaland				3
Burundi				2–6
Cameroon				20
Central Africa	Pygmies			4
Congo (Kinshasa)				6–23
Egypt				3·6
Ethiopia				0
Gambia				12–22
Ghana				14–24
Kenya				2–25
Libya				1
Madagascar				15
Nigeria	Yoruba	57	21	22
Nigeria				10–27
Ruanda				2–6
Senegal				5–12
South Africa				3–9
Southwest Africa	Bushmen			2–4
South Rhodesia				4–20
Swaziland				4
Uganda				15
Tanzania				2–28
Brazil	34% Negro	85	8	7
U.S.A.	Negro	70	18	12
Venezuela	Negro			11·5

The distribution of G-6-P D defect throughout the world is shown in Figure XVI, and the distribution in Africa in Figure XX. Table XLI gives figures for the incidence of the different variants of G-6-P D in various countries of Africa, Brazil, Venezuela and the United States (127).

XIX : Clinical Manifestations of
G-6-P D Deficiency

THE IMPORTANT manifestations of G-6-P D deficiency in Africans have been listed in Table XXXVII and include neonatal jaundice, hemolytic reactions during the course of infections, and hemolytic reactions following the administration of certain drugs. These reactions may be seen in the heterozygous female but are more likely to occur in the homozygous female or hemizygous male.

The drugs which are likely to provoke hemolysis are listed in Table XXXVIII (76). Although acetylsalicylic acid, aspirin, does not cause detectable hemolysis in doses of 4 grams daily, a dose of 10 grams may do so. With primaquine, 45 mg. daily causes severe hemolysis, 30 mg. daily moderate hemolysis and 15 mg. daily slight hemolysis. A dose of 45 mg. weekly, which is equivalent to $6\frac{1}{2}$ mg. daily, is well tolerated and effective against the exoerythrocytic phase of vivax malaria (3).

Some of the drugs listed in Table XXXVIII, namely phenylhydrazine, the sulfones, sulfathiazole and sulfapyridine may produce a hemolytic reaction in individuals with normal enzyme activity. However, in the presence of G-6-P D deficiency the hemolysis is likely to be more severe.

Certain metabolic disturbances such as hypoglycemia, diabetic acidosis, chronic renal disease or liver damage may aggravate the tendency towards hemolysis (76). Infections may bring on a hemolytic reaction and may aggravate the drug induced reaction. In the United States where there is widespread use of drugs, these only accounted for 40 per cent of the hemolytic reactions occurring in individuals with G-6-P D deficiency (169).

An important factor which tends to reduce the intensity towards hemolysis is the presence of an abnormally young population of red cells. Thus, the readministration of primaquine a week or two after a hemolytic reaction does not provoke hemolysis. It takes six to eight weeks for the red cell population to come back to normal (76). Some diseases are characterized by a permanent reticulocytosis. Thus, in sickle cell anemia and thalassemia the administration of potentially hemolytic drugs is less likely to cause a reaction. In fact, in these conditions it may be difficult to demonstrate deficiency of the enzyme G-6-P D even when the defect is inherited (87).

The hemolytic reaction which follows the administration of drugs can be divided into three phases, see Figure XLIII. These phases may

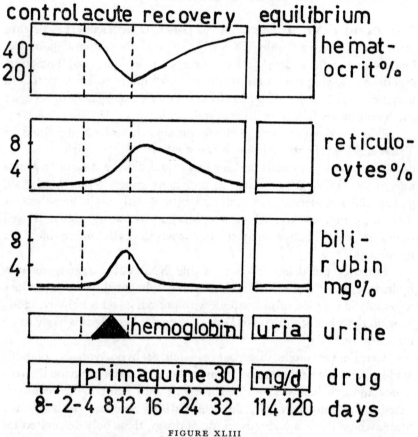

FIGURE XLIII
The three phases of primaquine hemolysis
Course of experimentally induced hemolytic anemia in primaquine-sensitive individual. (From Alving, A. S., *et al.*, Bull. World Health Org. **22**:621, 1960)

be detected whether the administration of the drug is continued or not. The first phase comes on about 48 hours after the administration of the drug and lasts for about a week. During this phase there is hemolysis of red cells with a fall in the hemoglobin level and hematocrit. There may be a liberation of hemoglobin into the plasma to such an extent that it appears in the urine giving it a dark colour. The increased serum level of hemoglobin causes a fall in serum haptoglobin. As the hemolysis progresses, icterus develops and the van den Bergh reaction shows a rise in both free and conjugated bilirubin. The urine may contain bilirubin as well as hemoglobin. With a daily dose of 30 mg. primaquine, half of the red cells may be hemolyzed and the total serum bilirubin level may exceed 10 mg. per 100 ml. The acute hemolytic phase may be accompanied by pain in the back and abdomen, weakness, and other symptoms of rapidly developing anemia. On the other hand the hemolytic reaction may go un-noticed (76).

The second phase of the hemolytic reaction is the recovery period when hemolysis stops, icterus fades and there is a marked reticulocytosis. This leads to a rise in the number of red cells and a restoration of the hemoglobin level towards normal. When the normal level is reached, it is said to be the third phase of the reaction or that of compensated anemia. Under these circumstances the reticulocyte count is slightly higher than normal and the red cell survival slightly reduced. These two factors balance out so that the hemoglobin level remains constant. In individuals with G-6-P D deficiency who have not been treated with any drugs the red cell survival is about 10 per cent shorter than in normals (98).

When a hemolytic reaction occurs during the administration of one of the drugs listed in Table XXXVIII the offending drug should be discontinued and if the anemia is severe transfusions may be required. Drugs which can provoke hemolysis in G-6-P D deficiency should be avoided in persons of African ancestry unless the enzyme defect has been ruled out by appropriate tests.

Neonatal jaundice of greater intensity than that which is deemed physiological occurs in association with G-6-P D defect in Greeks, Chinese and Africans (47) but has not been reported in full term Negro infants in the United States unless there is a history of drug administration, infection or prematurity (109). For this reason it is thought that environmental factors may be involved in the occurrence of neonatal jaundice in association with G-6-P D defect. This is most likely true because, even in Africa, only a small percentage of children born with G-6-P D defect develop neonatal jaundice.

The differential diagnosis between physiological jaundice, jaundice associated with G-6-P D defect, and jaundice due to ABO or Rh incompatibility is outlined in Table XLII. Physiological jaundice is seen a few days after birth, does not become intense, and rapidly disappears. Furthermore, there is no associated anemia, the red cells are normal, and there are few normoblasts. But when there is an associated G-6-P D deficiency, the jaundice may become more intense and last for a longer time. Peculiarly enough, the onset of jaundice in these cases is not earlier than in the case of physiological jaundice. If either the mother or child is given large doses of vitamin K there is a greater likelihood of the development of jaundice (174). When the jaundice is associated with G-6-P D deficiency, there may be an associated anemia (45).

TABLE XLII

DIFFERENTIAL DIAGNOSIS OF EARLY NEONATAL JAUNDICE

Diagnosis	Physio-logical jaundice	G-6-P D defect	ABO incompati-bility	Rh incompati-bility
van den Bergh	indirect	indirect	indirect	indirect
Daily increment of over 5 mg.%	no	yes	yes	yes
Maximum level	12 mg.%	variable	variable	variable
Day of onset	2–3	3–5	0–1	1–2
Day of maximum	3–4	variable	variable	variable
Day disappearance	4–7	variable	variable	variable
Mother's blood group and enzyme	variable	G-6-P D defect	O group	Rh negative
Child's blood group and enzyme	variable	G-6-P D defect	A or B	Rh positive
Direct Coombs test	negative	negative	negative	positive
Indir. Coombs test	negative	negative	positive	positive
Parity of mother	variable	variable	variable	high
Size of RBC	normal	normal	small	large
Anemia	none	moderate	slight	moderate
Normoblasts	few	moderate	moderate	many
Kernicterus	none	rare	rare	frequent
Stillbirth	none	none	none	occasional

Erythroblastosis fetalis due to Rh incompatibility is not as common in Africa as in Europe and America because of the relatively much smaller proportion of Rh negative individuals. In the differential diagnosis, jaundice due to blood incompatibility is likely to occur earlier than in physiological jaundice or jaundice associated with G-6-P D deficiency. In ABO incompatibility the red cells are likely to be smaller than normal and there is little anemia while in Rh incompatibility the cells are larger than normal and the anemia may be severe. Although Rh incompatibility is a severe type of reaction it does not usually affect the first pregnancies as it takes time for the antibodies to Rh to build up (53). On the other hand, jaundice associated with G-6-P D deficiency may affect the first and subsequent deliveries to the same extent.

Most cases of jaundice associated with G-6-P D defect subside spontaneously, but if the serum bilirubin level rises above 25 mg. per 100 ml. there is the possibility of cerebral damage as well as a threat to life (45). In such cases exchange transfusion is indicated.

Jaundice associated with G-6-P D deficiency is a frequent occurrence in some types of infection. Viral hepatitis produces more jaundice than usual when there is associated G-6-P D deficiency (29) (139). Pneumonia may cause hemolysis in normal individuals and this may be more intense in patients with G-6-P D deficiency. Another infection, common in the tropics, which may cause a hemolytic reaction in G-6-P D deficient subjects is typhoid fever (162).

Despite the theoretical protection against malaria that has been postulated for individuals with G-6-P D deficiency, children with the enzyme deficiency are more prone to develop anemia as a result of chronic malaria infection than children with normal enzyme activity (70).

XX : Treatment of Sickle Cell Disease

TREATMENT in sickle cell disease may be directed at an improvement of the steady state and the prevention of crises or complications. On the other hand, treatment is sometimes required for crises or complications. Treatment of pregnancy in sickle cell disease has been discussed in Chapter XIV.

To improve the steady state and prevent the occurrence of crises and complications, it is advisable to promote good nutrition and to avoid any stresses or strains. A special effort is required to prevent any type of infection and to render prompt treatment when prophylaxis fails.

The nutrition of the individual with sickle cell disease differs from that of the average person in that there is a greater requirement for folic acid which is required to support the high rate of erythropoesis (91) (167). Hence dietary supplements of up to 5 mg. folic acid daily are often prescribed, especially in areas where folic acid deficiency may occur. Although such treatment is not always necessary or beneficial (116) it is not associated with any possibility of harmful effect. In fact folic acid has become the standard placebo treatment for sickle cell disease. However, in the presence of megaloblastosis, folic acid is of proven value (167).

Despite the high rate of turnover of iron, the individual with sickle cell disease does not seem to be prone to the development of iron deficiency. Furthermore, this high rate of turnover and the occasional need for transfusions renders the patient with sickle cell anemia liable to the development of hemosiderosis (128). For these reasons and because of lack of effectiveness, iron salts are only occasionally employed in the treatment of sickle cell disease (144).

In sickle cell disease, there is usually a certain degree of anemia which has been explained on the basis that the shift in oxygen dissociation curve allows the tissues an abundance of oxygen despite the reduced level (12). However, when the hemoglobin level falls below 8 grams in sickle cell anemia or below 11 grams in sickle cell hemoglobin C disease, blood transfusions may be given. In fact some investigators remove a small volume of the patient's blood and replace it with normal blood in a program of partial exchange transfusion (5). Prior to elective surgery, or in the treatment of cutaneous ulcers, transfusions may be used to bring the hemoglobin up to a normal level, thus suppressing the formation of red cells by the patient (28) (38). Repeated transfusions are not without hazard, especially in sickle cell disease. There is the possibility of transmitting viral hepatitis, of inducing iron overload, and of causing a transfusion reaction. In addition, transfusion may initiate a serious or fatal crisis in sickle cell disease (113).

Methods required for the prophylaxis of infections in patients with sickle cell disease depend upon the environmental hazards as well as the age of the individual. For the infant, the usual vaccinations should be carried out including BCG, measles, diphtheria, pertussis, tetanus and poliomyelitis. Gamma globulin may be used as prophylaxis against hepatitis in areas where the disease is common. In view of the frequency of salmonella infections at all ages (118), repeated immunization against typhoid and paratyphoid is advisable. On principle, prophylaxis with antibiotics should be avoided, unless there are specific indications, because of the danger of inducing sensitivity in the patient and resistance in the micro-organisms. There is ample evidence from long term trials conducted in East (165) and West (58) Africa that malaria chemo-prophylaxis improves the general condition and reduces the incidence of crises. In fact, some of the benefits ascribed to folic acid (167) and the combination of promazine and dapsone (84) may have been due to the antimalarial chemoprophylaxis. It appears that the most effective drug, at least in West Africa, is chloroquine (58). Adults and grown children should be given 400 mg. of the sulfate or 500 mg. of the phosphate at weekly intervals while smaller children can be given half this dose and infants a quarter. Long term treatment with anti-coagulants is dangerous (140) and since the role of acidosis in spontaneous crises has not been proven (61) the use of alkali salts as a routine measure is questionable.

The treatment of crises and complications is a different matter. Here, transfusions are of immediate and marked benefit in the aplastic and the hemolytic type of crisis. Those patients with hemolytic crises associated with hypersplenism are markedly benefited by splenectomy (40) (89) (154). Adrenal cortical hormone may be given prior to the operation as this leads to a reduction in the size of the spleen (89).

Painful crises are of such variability that it is difficult to assess treatment. Transfusions should be avoided unless there are special indications but parenteral fluid is required. Alkali salts give the same results as normal saline (143). Dextran likewise gives the same results

TABLE XLIII

THERAPEUTIC PROCEDURES IN SICKLE CELL DISEASE

Treatment	Steady state	Hemolytic crises	Aplastic crises	Painful crises
Immunization	+			
Antibiotics	+			
Antimalarials	+			
Folic acid	+	+	+	
Transfusions	+	+	+	
Alkali salts	+			+
Dextran				+
Plasma				+
Saline				+
Analgesics				+
Narcotics				+
Phenothiazines				+

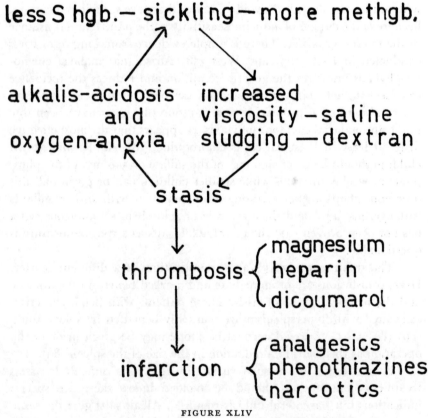

FIGURE XLIV

The vicious cycle of sickling and therapeutic approaches

as normal saline (9) (111). In mild cases analgesics such as acetylsalicylic acid or paracetamol may be sufficient to control pain but in severe cases pethidine (demerol) is often required. Since this is an addictive drug, there is some advantage to using a tranquilizer such as promazine. The latter will allay the pains and allow the patient to sleep. In mild cases it can be given orally, in more severe cases intramuscularly, and in very severe cases by slow intravenous injection (84). This drug is also useful in allaying the symptoms in infants with hand foot syndrome. On the other hand, long term treatment with small doses of promazine does not reduce the incidence of painful episodes (110). Nevertheless promazine, chlorpromazine and promethazine (138) have often been used in the management of sickle cell disease.

There is no specific therapy for complications involving the eyes or the skeletal system. Rest, sedation and symptomatic treatment are indicated. Infections should be uncovered and treated. Folic acid and antimalarials are indicated. Anticoagulants and antibiotics may be given when there is evidence of thrombophlebitis (88).

Methemoglobin formation retards the sickling process (16). When induced by sodium nitrite severe headache is produced. When induced

TABLE XLIV

THERAPY FOR COMPLICATIONS OF SICKLE CELL DISEASE

Complication	Treatment used
Anemia	Transfusion
	Folic acid
Hypersplenism	Adrenal cortical hormone
	Transfusions
	Splenectomy
Hematuria	Transfusion
Aseptic necrosis	Immobilization
Osteomyelitis	Antibiotics
Hand foot syndrome	Analgesics
	Phenothiazines
Priapism	Sodium lactate
	Phenothiazines
Vitreous and retinal hemorrhage	Alkali salts
Marrow embolism	Heparin
Phlebitis	Dicoumarol
Cutaneous ulcers	Transfusion
	Immobilization
Abdominal crises and splenic infarct	Sodium lactate
	Phenothiazines
Epistaxis	Vitamin K

with dapsone, there are no symptoms but the level may not be high enough to be of benefit.

The therapeutic procedures that have been used in sickle cell disease are summarized in Table XLIII and their rationale portrayed in Figure XLIV. Measures that can be taken when complications occur are given in Table XLIV.

XXI : Public Health Aspects of Sickle Cell Disease

IN A DISCUSSION of the social aspects of sickle cell disease, one can include the provision of laboratory services, the operation of blood banks, the estimation of the occupational ability of individuals with abnormal hemoglobin diseases, the morbidity and mortality of these diseases and finally the advisability of genetic counseling. Many of these public health aspects are inter-related.

The two most important laboratory tests which are needed, the sickling test (142) and the paper electrophoretic analysis (93) are described in subsequent chapters. In hospital centers, especially those with a large maternity service, it may be useful to test for G-6-P D deficiency (127). This test is also described in a subsequent chapter. It may be necessary for the public health services to inaugurate or supervise these laboratory procedures.

In smaller laboratories, it may be convenient to perform the sickling test and to forward to a larger center samples of blood for the electrophoretic test. In this case, efficient organization is required to insure accurate results and prompt reporting.

Most blood banks measure the hemoglobin level of prospective donors and take a brief history to make sure that the donor does not have an illness which would endanger either the donor or the recipient. This simple routine will eliminate most individuals with sickle cell anemia, who have a hemoglobin level well below normal, and most individuals with sickle cell hemoglobin C disease, who usually give a history of having suffered from rheumatic pains. However, this procedure would not eliminate individuals with sickle cell trait or G-6-P D deficiency. Fortunately, blood from such individuals is suitable for transfusion (75). The only exception to this rule is in the case of exchange transfusions when it is inadvisable to use blood from individuals with G-6-P D deficiency or sickle cell trait (163). When the blood bank takes a sample for the measurement of the hemoglobin level, or for typing, it would not entail much extra time or expense to perform a sickling test. When the sickling test is positive an electrophoretic analysis can be requested. The blood donor is entitled to receive information as to his blood group and as to the presence or absence of sickling. This information can be entered on a durable card which the donor can keep for future reference.

Sickling tests should be performed on all pregnant women, individuals who are to undergo major surgical procedures, and on pediatric or medical cases that present with anemia. In such cases the results of the test can be kept in the patient's case history and entered on a durable card as recommended for the blood bank.

With respect to occupational ability, individuals with G-6-P D deficiency do not suffer from any occupational handicap, and people with sickle cell trait are only at risk when the type of work entails frequent exposure to reduced oxygen pressure (74). Although there are military and civilian pilots who have sickle cell trait, and who have not suffered from any disability during their career, there is still some risk involved, especially that of splenic infarct (134). It is, therefore, advisable to discourage individuals with sickle cell trait from entering a career which involves frequent airplane flights. On the other hand, it is not necessary to dismiss or ground individuals who have already been trained or employed before the sickling trait was noted. These individuals deserve the benefit of medical supervision.

The presence of sickle cell disease renders the candidate unfit for frequent airplane flights and such persons should be exempted from military or naval service unless a sedentary position is insured. Individuals with sickle cell disease should avoid jobs which entail heavy labour or frequent exposure to inclement weather. Light labour and occasional exposure to variable weather can be tolerated by most patients with sickle cell hemoglobin C disease and a few of the patients with sickle cell anemia. But for some individuals with sickle cell hemoglobin C disease and most with sickle cell anemia it is advisable to seek employment limited to sedentary work, see Table XLV (84).

The morbidity and mortality of sickle cell disease depends on the particular individual and on his environment. As economic, social and medical conditions improve the outlook becomes brighter. In some parts of Africa, adults with sickle cell anemia are rare, and most of the children with sickle cell anemia succumb before reaching maturity (80). In other parts of Africa (84), in the West Indies (4) (144), and in the United States (26), the prognosis is better. The age distribution of individuals with sickle cell anemia is contrasted with that of an analogous population in Figure XLV (26). However, there is still a high morbidity and a need for medical supervision, preferably in clinics

TABLE XLV

OCCUPATIONAL ABILITY AND SICKLE CELL DISEASE*

Occupational ability	Sickle cell anemia	Sickle cell hemoglobin C disease	Sickle cell trait	G-6-P D defect
Civilian or military air services	—	—	—	+
Naval or military services	—	—	+	+
Heavy or out-door labour	—	—	+	+
Light or in-door labour	—	+	+	+
Sedentary work	+	+	+	+

* Sickle cell thalassemia occupies a position intermediate between sickle cell anemia and sickle cell hemoglobin C disease. Some such individuals have the same capacity as patients with sickle cell hemoglobin C disease while others are as limited as patients with sickle cell anemia.

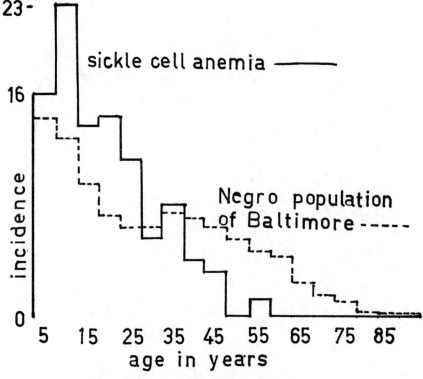

FIGURE XLV

Age distribution of 100 proved cases of sickle cell anemia, compared with that of the Negro population of Baltimore.

especially designed for the care of individuals with sickle cell disease or hematological problems.

It has been suggested that individuals with sickle cell trait should be discouraged from selecting a partner with sickle cell trait. And when such marriages take place, the number of children should be limited. Academically minded geneticists have pointed out that the incidence of the S gene is kept in check by mating between pairs with sickle cell trait and that interference with this means of natural selection is disadvantageous to the general population. However, good medical care also interferes with this process of natural selection. Regardless of the theoretical considerations, individuals deserve to know the risk involved in bearing and rearing children with sickle cell disease. If both partners have sickle cell trait, there is a 25 per cent chance that each child will have sickle cell disease, and the risk is not altered by the previous birth of "sicklers" or normal children.

XXII : Sickling Tests

AT TIMES, sickled red blood cells may be found in the circulating blood (59) but at other times there may be no evidence of sickling so that the absence of sickled forms has no diagnostic significance while the presence of sickled forms suggests sickle cell disease. On the other hand, when blood from patients with sickle cell disease or individuals with sickle cell trait is allowed to deoxygenate spontaneously, or is reduced by artificial means, the sickled cells appear (41). If the degree of oxygen deprivation can be accurately controlled it is possible to distinguish between sickle cell anemia and sickle cell trait but the variants of sickle cell disease have an intermediate status (145).

Deoxygenation and sickling can be hastened by the addition of methylene blue (52) or a variety of reducing agents such as ascorbic acid and sodium metabisulfite (35). Another technique for accelerating deoxygenation is the addition of a pure culture of colon bacilli or a ten per cent suspension of fecal matter in normal saline (96). Sickling is accelerated by raising the temperature from that of the laboratory to that of the body (145).

A drop of blood taken from the finger may be tested for sickling without the addition of any anticoagulant. If there is some delay before the test can be carried out, the blood should be prevented from coagulating by the addition of heparin, citrate or ethylenediamine-tetra acetic acid (171). Sterile precautions are required when blood is taken for shipment to another laboratory, unless there are facilities to keep the blood cool during transportation. Similarly blood may be stored in a refrigerator but should not be kept indefinitely at room temperature before the sickling test is carried out.

The first stage of sickling, *in vivo* or *in vitro* is the formation of a single point projecting from the red cell membrane. Subsequently there may be narrowing and elongation of the cell with additional points appearing usually at opposite ends of the cell but sometimes only at one end. If the points are distributed around the cell it takes on a holly leaf shape. If the points are on one side there is a brush-like appearance. Elongated, two-pointed cells look like an oat grain and when such a cell is curved it has the shape of a banana. The most extreme form of sickling is manifested by the appearance of long thread-like processes from one or more of the points. Some of these cells may resemble a sickle. Figure XLVI shows several of the forms which should be distinguished from crenated red cells as shown in Figure VIII (34).

The most rapid and accurate method for obtaining a simple positive or negative sickling test is to take a drop of blood, place it on a clean slide and add 2–3 drops of a freshly prepared solution of 2 per cent sodium metabisulfite. The blood and the solution are mixed with the corner of a clean cover slip which is then placed on top of the blood mixture. Excess blood is removed with a piece of filter, tissue or blotting paper so that a thin film of blood lies between the two layers of glass. The slide may be inspected immediately and if sickling is noted a positive result can be reported. If no sickling is seen the slide should be kept for an hour and then inspected again. If the air is dry the slide can be kept in a moist chamber or sealed. A final report can be made after 1 hour. Too high a concentration of sodium metabisulfite can give a false positive result (142). More important, if the sodium metabisulfite has deteriorated due to exposure to heat or moisture, or if the solution has been prepared on a previous day, a false negative result may be obtained. Other factors which may cause misleading results are listed in Table XLVI (158). A convenient technique is to keep the sodium

TABLE XLVI
CAUSES OF ERROR IN THE SICKLING TESTS

Type of test	False positives	False negatives
Moist test and $Na_2S_2O_5$ test	Transfusion with sickle trait blood	Deterioration of blood sample (hemolysis)
	Presence of poikilocytosis or eliptocytosis	High concentration F Hgb.*
	Drying of film at the edges	Insufficient time or searching
$Na_2S_2O_5$ test only	Too high a concentration $Na_2S_2O_5$	Deterioration of $Na_2S_2O_5$
Moist test		G-6-P D deficiency
		Administration of dapsone
		Too low a room temperature

* Especially in cord blood, blood from young infants and in the rare condition of persistent fetal hemoglobin gene.

metabisulfite in packets of 200 mg. in a desiccator or tightly sealed jar and to empty the contents into 10 ml. of distilled water just before performing the test.

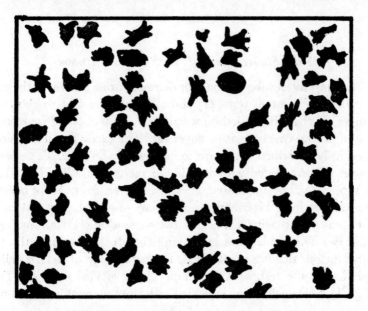

sickle cell trait

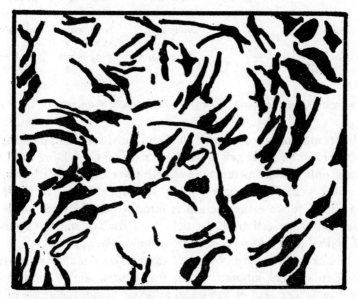

sickle cell anemia

FIGURE XLVI

Sickling in a sealed preparation

Photomicrograph of sickled red cells

Hb-S trait. A similar preparation to that shown above. "Holly-leaf" sickling is shown. ×900.

Photomicrograph of sickled red cells

Sealed preparation of blood. Hb-S disease. Fully sickled filamentous forms predominate. ×900.

From: *Practical Haematology* by Dacie and Lewis

The most interesting method for demonstrating sickling is the moist test, called the Emmel test (41) since he was the first to show that "cultures" of red cells sickled on standing. A drop of blood is placed on a clean slide and covered with a cover slip. The excess blood is removed as previously described with care to exclude air bubbles. The edges of the cover slip are sealed with vaseline or melted paraffin. The slide is then kept at 25° or incubated at 37° for three days. More constant results are obtained if sterile precautions are observed. This test can be used to make a tentative distinction between sickle cell trait and sickle cell disease. The guide lines in making this distinction are: the time required before sickling is observed, the percentage of sickled cells on completion of the test, and the shape of the sickled cells, see Table XLVII. In sickle cell anemia, sickled cells are seen within a few hours,

TABLE XLVII

USUAL RESULTS OBTAINED WITH MOIST SICKLING TEST*

Criterion	Normal persons	Sickle cell trait	Sickle cell HGB C	Sickle cell anemia
Form of red cells	disc	holly leaf	holly leaf or oat	filamentous
Time for sickling	—	6–72 hours	3–24 hours	0–12 hours
Percentage sickling 24 hours	0	1–50	25–75	50–100

* The figures given here vary according to the details of the test.

at 24 hours most of the cells are sickled, and the sickled cells show thread-like extensions. In sickle cell trait, there may be no sickling until after 12 hours, only a small percentage of cells are sickled at 24 hours, and most of the sickled cells have a holly leaf appearance. In sickle cell hemoglobin C disease the picture is intermediate between sickle cell anemia and sickle cell trait. In sickle cell thalassemia the course of events is similar to that seen in sickle cell anemia.

The sickle test requires care and experience. An analysis of results obtained in clinical laboratories in the United States showed false positives in 25 per cent of cases and an even higher incidence of false negatives (158). A false positive result may be due to a transfusion of sickle cell trait blood given within the previous three months. Ellipto-cytosis and poikilocytosis may lead to confusion. A false negative test may be obtained when there is a high concentration of fetal hemo-globin. This is especially likely to occur in cord blood so that special techniques are used in such cases. A sodium metabisulfite test is made, the preparation is sealed and the final reading is made after 24 hours of incubation.

When the sodium metabisulfite test is employed, the laboratory can only report sickling positive or sickling negative. If the Emmel test is used, the laboratory can report the time required before sickling takes place, the percentage of sickled cells at 24 hours, and the form of sickling that is observed. This information may assist the clinician who has already formed a clinical impression. However, the Emmel test is subject to great variation (123) and there are limitations in its interpretation. An electrophoresis is required for a definitive diagnosis.

If blood from a patient is sickle positive, it is valuable to test the blood of both parents. If both parents show sickling the patient may have sickle cell trait or sickle cell anemia, but cannot have sickle cell hemoglobin C disease or sickle cell thalassemia unless one of the parents has these illnesses. If one of the parents shows sickling and the other does not, then sickle cell anemia is ruled out and the patient may have sickle cell trait, sickle cell hemoglobin C disease or sickle cell hemoglobin D disease or sickle cell thalassemia.

XXIII : Zone Electrophoresis

ELECTROPHORETIC separation of hemoglobin was discovered by Pauling in 1949 (115). Subsequently zone electrophoresis on paper was developed as a routine laboratory method (72). The requirements for this method of hemoglobin separation are a supporting medium, a buffer solution, and an apparatus to hold the supporting medium and buffer, and through which a suitable electric current passes, see Table XLVIII (93).

TABLE XLVIII

ZONE ELECTROPHORESIS OF HEMOGLOBIN

Supporting medium	Buffer used		Apparatus used
Whatman No. 1	Barbiturate	8·9	Horizontal
Whatman No. 3 for	Tris buffer	8·9	
chromatography	Phosphate	6.5	
Whatman No. 100 for	Barbiturate	8·9	Vertical
chromatography	Tris buffer	8·9	
Whatman 3 MM	Phosphate	6·5	
Cellulose acetate	Barbiturate	8·9	Horizontal
Starch gel	Tris buffer	8·9	
Agar gel	Phosphate	6·5	

The simplest supporting medium is filter paper or cellulose acetate paper. For more accurate separations, agar gel or starch block may be used as a supporting medium. The cellulose acetate paper has the advantage of giving more rapid results. The filter paper electrophoresis is quite versatile and can be used with either a horizontal or vertical electrophoresis apparatus (181).

Various buffers have been employed, see Table XLIX. Barbiturate buffer at pH 8·6–8·9 is satisfactory for separating the three most common West African hemoglobins, A, S, and C. Tris buffer at pH 8·9 is useful for separating A_2 from A which helps in the diagnosis of thalassemia trait (49). Phosphate buffer at pH 6·5 is used to separate S and D hemoglobins which migrate at the same rate in alkaline buffer (93).

The first step in zone electrophoresis is the preparation of the hemoglobin sample. This is a chemically pure solution containing about 10 per cent of hemoglobin in distilled water. The hemoglobin is

TABLE XLIX

COMPOSITION OF BUFFERS FOR ZONE ELECTROPHORESIS

Barbiturate buffer 8·9 for separating A, S, and C.

sodium diethylbarbiturate	10·3 grams
diethylbarbituric acid	0·92 grams
distilled water to	1 liter

Tris buffer 8·9 for separating A_2 and A

tris-(hydroxymethyl)-amino methane	50·4 grams
ethylenediamine-tetra-acetic acid	5·0 grams
boric acid	3·8 grams
distilled water to	1 liter

Phosphate buffer 6·5 for separating S and D

sodium dihydrogen phosphate	0·587 grams
disodium hydrogen phosphate	1·49 grams
distilled water to	1 liter

obtained by hemolysis of the red cells which can be accomplished by freezing and thawing one volume of red cells in two volumes of water. Better results are obtained if the cells are washed and freed of lipoid material. According to this scheme a sample of blood is taken and mixed with an anticoagulant. The blood is then centrifuged and the plasma removed by suction. The red cells are then resuspended in four times their volume of normal saline, remixed and respun. The saline is removed by suction and the process repeated twice. Then the red cells are suspended in one and a half volumes of distilled water plus a half volume of carbon tetrachloride. This time the centrifuge tube is corked with a rubber stopper and shaken for 5 minutes. The mixture is centrifuged and the pure hemoglobin solution, which lies at the top, is ready for electrophoresis. The pure solution may be stored at 4° C. until ready for use (81).

The next step is to prepare the filter paper for the application of the hemoglobin solution. The paper is held with a forceps to prevent contamination by the fingers. The paper should be kept free from moisture and stored in a cool place, but not in a refrigerator. Individual strips 1 inch wide or a broad strip with several samples can be used. The paper should be gently marked with a lead pencil in a line perpendicular to the strip at the center(93).

Approximately 0·01 ml. of the hemoglobin solution is applied on the pencil line using a capillary pipette or a camel hair brush. The line of application must be straight and the pipette should be held perpendicular to the surface of the paper. Then the paper is moistened by dipping the ends into the buffer compartments of the electrode bath of the electrophoretic apparatus. Additional fresh buffer is applied to the suspended paper by means of a pipette, but in such a manner as the moisture approaches the line of hemoglobin from both sides simultaneously (72).

With cellulose acetate paper it is necessary to moisten the strips before the application of the hemoglobin. After making the pencil mark the paper is moistened and blotted and then the hemoglobin solution is applied.

During electrophoresis the strips and electrode compartments are kept covered to prevent evaporation. Since heat is developed during the electrophoresis it is preferable to place the apparatus in an air-conditioned room or refrigerator.

In the horizontal apparatus, the paper is supported by strips of perspex and the ends of the paper dip into the inner buffer troughs that connect by a porous device with the outer buffer troughs which hold the platinum wire electrodes. The current used is approximately 0·75 milliamperes per inch width of paper at a potential of 250 volts. With such a system, the separation requires 16–20 hours.

In the vertical apparatus, see Figure XLVII, the strips are hung over a perspex bar and the ends dip into the inner troughs of the electrophoresis apparatus. A similar current will give good separation in the same time as with the horizontal method although slightly more current is required with barbiturate buffer as compared with tris buffer.

The advantage of cellulose acetate paper is the greater rapidity of the method, but only the horizontal type of apparatus can be used. A current of 1 milliampere per inch of paper at the same voltage will produce separation of the hemoglobins in approximately four hours (93).

The same buffer can be used for several runs if the polarity of the bath is reversed with each run. Nevertheless, fresh buffer must be prepared from time to time. The efficiency of separation can be checked by including a sample of sickle cell trait or hemoglobin C trait blood with each run.

A "power pack" unit is furnished with most electrophoresis tanks which makes it possible to deliver a variable cirrent at a fixed voltage, the current being adjusted to the number of strips in the tank.

After the electrophoretic separation has been completed the strips can be dried in a current of warm air or in an oven at 100°C. The hemoglobin spots are self evident so that staining is not required.

If the hemoglobin sample has to be sent to a distant laboratory for electrophoresis, the sample should be collected with sterile technique or

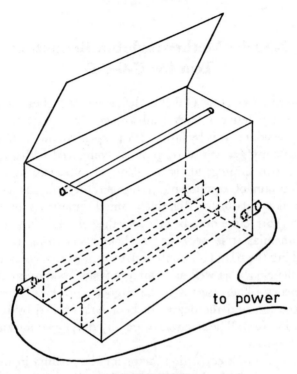

FIGURE XLVII
Apparatus for zone electrophoresis
Vertical tank for paper electrophoresis. The tank is constructed from Perspex with a nylon string for supporting the papers. The top plate is of plate glass as Perspex plates tend to buckle. 45 × 17 × 23 cm. Similar apparatus is available through Amer Products, 56 Rochester Place, London N.W.1.
From: *Chromatographic and Electrophoretique Techniques* Edited by Ivor Smith.

refrigerated during transit. If the plasma has been removed and the red cells have been washed, hemolysis during transport will not affect the results (152).

XXIV : Methemoglobin Reduction
Test for G-6-P D

THERE are many tests for G-6-P D deficiency (15), but the methemo-globin reduction test has several advantages (20) (21). It is a simple and rapid procedure. It is by far the least expensive method, consuming less than a penny's worth of reagents as compared with prepackaged tests costing two shillings for each assay. The test can be carried out with a minimum of equipment, a refrigerator and incubator being useful but not necessary. Relatively small quantities of blood are required. No correction need be made for the hemoglobin level although in severe anemias it is necessary to hemoconcentrate the specimen before running the test. This method detects most cases of heterozygous or partial deficiency as well as hemizygous and homozygous or com-plete deficiency. There seems to be a good correlation between the results of the test and the degree of hemolysis evoked by primaquine administration (21). The test was originally developed for and used on American Negroes.

The absence of a correction factor for the anemia in the calcula-tion of results obviates the false normal reading obtained with the quantitative test when applied to individuals with hemolytic anemias (87).

The principle on which the methemoglobin reduction test is based is that the enzyme G-6-P D enhances the formation of NADPH (TPNH). This byproduct of the enzyme reaction in turn enhances the activity of the NADPH-dependent methemoglobin reductase. In the test, hemo-globin is converted by the nitrite ion to methemoglobin. The glucose and methylene blue favour the action of G-6-P D. The NADPH is required for the reduction of methemoglobin to hemoglobin. In the normal person, this process is completed in two hours. When there is partial deficiency of G-6-P D the process takes 4–8 hours while with complete deficiency it may take up to 24 hours. Instead of measuring the time required for complete regeneration of hemoglobin, the percen-tage not regenerated in 3 hours is estimated. The finding of 100 per cent methemoglobin does not mean that there is no activity, see Table XXXIV (127).

Under no circumstances should oxalate mixtures be used to prevent coagulation of the blood as oxalates interfere with enzyme activity (21). Either heparin, citrate or ethylenediamine-tetra-acetate can be used. The best anticoagulant for this purpose is ACD solution, as the blood can be kept in the cold for several days without loss of activity. This solution contains 2·45 gm. dextrose, 0·80 gm. citric acid and 2·20 gm. trisodium citrate per 100 ml. of distilled water. An amount of 0·15 ml. of this solution is sufficient to prevent the coagulation of 1 ml. of blood.

The first reagent contains 1·25 gm. of sodium nitrite per 100 ml. of distilled water. However, if heparin or EDTA is used in place of ACD solution it is necessary to add 5·0 gm. glucose to this reagent.

The second reagent contains 0·15 gm. of trihydrated methylene blue chloride per 100 ml. of distilled water.

The reagents should be prepared once a month and if possible stored in a refrigerator. The sodium nitrite should be protected from intense light.

The procedure for the test involves setting up of two control test tubes, one for hemoglobin and one for methemoglobin, and a series of test tubes, one for each blood sample to be tested, see Figure XLVIII. These test tubes should have a diameter of 10–15 mm. and a height of 10–15 cm. With a pipettte, 0·1 ml. of the sodium nitrite reagent is placed in the methemoglobin tube and each of the tubes for testing blood samples. With another pipette 0·1 ml. of the methylene blue reagent is placed in the hemoglobin tube and each of the tubes for testing blood samples. Then 2 ml. of each blood sample is placed in its test tube and 2 ml. of any blood sample in the hemoglobin and methemoglobin tubes. Then the tubes are placed in an incubator for 3 hours. Following incubation the tubes are shaken and 0·1 ml. from each tube is placed in 10 ml. of water and shaken. After an interval of a few minutes to permit hemolysis, the tubes are inspected in daylight against a white background. The tube with sodium nitrite will contain only methemoglobin while the tube with methylene blue will contain only hemoglobin. The other tubes will contain hemoglobin, methemoglobin or a mixture of the two. When there is a mixture the percentage of methemoglobin can be estimated by comparing the tube with a 50 per cent mixture obtained by adding 5 ml. of the methemoglobin hemolysate to 5 ml. of the hemoglobin hemolysate.

If no methemoglobin is detected in a sample it may be assumed that the level of G-6-P D is normal or elevated, if only methemoglobin is seen it may be assumed that there is complete defect compatible with hemizygous or homozygous deficiency. On the other hand, if there is a

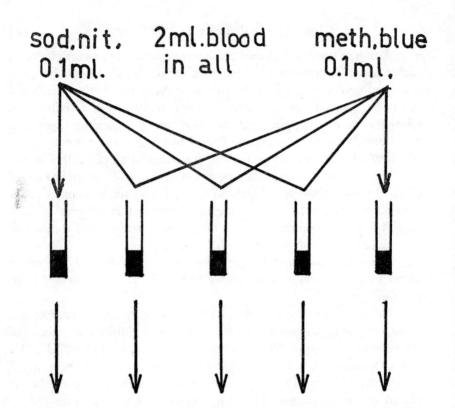

sod.nit.
0.1ml.

2ml.blood
in all

meth.blue
0.1ml.

incubated 3 hours, diluted 1/100

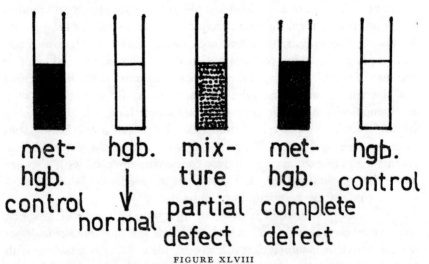

met-
hgb.
control

hgb.

↓

normal

mix-
ture

partial
defect

met-
hgb.
complete
defect

hgb.
control

FIGURE XLVIII
Flow sheet and reading of the methemoglobin reduction test

mixture of hemoglobin and methemoglobin it may be assumed that there is partial defect compatible with heterozygous deficiency. Partial defect does not occur in males unless there is an inherited complete defect modified by hemolytic anemia causing an enhanced enzyme activity (141). The test has to be modified if hemoglobin H is present (131).

The test can be carried out with smaller volumes of blood. In this event, the two reagents are mixed in equal amounts and a volume equal to one tenth of the volume of blood is added before incubation. The incubated mixture is then diluted to ten times its volume with distilled water. The test has also been modified in such a manner as to be applicable to blood smears where it is possible to distinguish two populations of red cells in female heterozygotes (144).

References

1. ALLISON, A. C. (1956). Sickle Cell Anaemia and Haemoglobin C., *Trans. Roy. Soc. Trop. Med. Hyg.*, **50**: 185.
2. ALLISON, A. C., ASKONAS, B. A., BARNICOT, N. A., BLUMBERG, B. S. and KRIMBAS, C. (1963). Deficiency of Erythrocyte Glucose-6-Phosphate Dehydrogenase in Greek Populations, *Ann. Human Genet.*, **26**: 237.
3. ALVING, A. S., JOHNSON, C. F., TARLOV, A. B., KELLERMEYER, R. W., BREWER, G. J. and CARSON, P. E. (1960). Mitigation of the Haemolytic Effect of Primaquine and Enhancement of its Action Against Exoerythrocytic Forms of the Chesson Strain of *Plasmodium vivax* by Intermittent Regimens of Drug Administration, *Bull. Wld. Hlth. Org.*, **22**: 621.
4. ANDERSON, M., WENT, L. N., McIVER, J. E. and DIXON, H. G. (1960). Sickle Cell Disease in Pregnancy, *Lancet*, **2**: 516.
5. ANDERSON, R., CASSEL, M., MULLINAX, G. L. and CHAPLIN, H. Jr. (1963). Effect of Normal Cells on the Viscosity of Sickle Cell Blood: *In Vitro* Studies and Report on Six Years Experience with a Prophylactic Program of "Partial Exchange Transfusion", *Arch. Int. Med.*, **111**: 286.
6. APTHORP, G. H., MEASDAY, B. and LEHMANN, H. (1963). Pregnancy in Sickle Cell Anaemia, *Lancet*, **1**: 1344.
7. ARGEN, R. J. and SULLIVAN, M. A. (1966). Bone Changes in Sickle Cell Disease, *New York J. Med.*, **66**: 1238.
8. BAIRD, R. L., WEISS, D. L., FERGUSON, A. D., FRENCH, J. H. and SCOTT, R. B. (1964). Studies in Sickle Cell Anemia XXI Clinico-Pathological Aspects of Neurological Manifestations, *Pediat.*, **34**: 92.
9. BARNES, P. M., HENDRICKSE, R. G. and WATSON-WILLIAMS, E. J. (1965). Low Molecular Weight Dextran in Treatment of Bone Pain Crises in Sickle Cell Disease: A Double Blind Trial, *Lancet*, **2**: 1271.
10. BARRERAS, L. and DIGGS, L. W. (1964). Bicarbonates, pH and Percentage of Sickled Cells in Venous Blood of Patients in Sickle Cell Crisis, *Am. J. Med. Sci.*, **247**: 710.
11. BASU, A. K. and WOODRUFF, A. W. (1966). Effect of Acetazolamide and Magnesium Therapy on Erythrocyte Survival in Sickle Cell Anaemia and Sickle Cell Haemoglobin C Disease, *Trans. Roy. Soc. Trop. Med. Hyg.*, **60**: 64.
12. BELLINGHAM, A. J. and HUEHNS, E. R. (1968). Compensation in Haemolytic Anaemias Caused by Abnormal Haemoglobins, *Nature*, **218**: 924.
13. BENNETT, M. A., HESLOP, R. W. and MEYNELL, M. J. (1967). Massive Haematuria Associated with Sickle-Cell Trait, *Brit. Med. J.*, **1**: 677.
14. BEUTLER, E. (1966). Abnormalities of Glycolysis (HMP Shunt) XI Cong. Internat. Soc. Haematol. Blight, Sydney.
15. BEUTLER, E. (1967). Glucose-6-Phosphate Dehydrogenase Deficiency, Diagnosis, Clinical and Genetic Implications, *Am. J. Clin. Path.*, **47**: 303.
16. BEUTLER, E. and MIKUS, B. J. (1961). Effect of Methemoglobin Formation in Sickle Cell Disease, *J. Clin. Invest.*, **40**: 1856.
17. BICKERS, J. N. (1966). Alkali Resistant Hemoglobin in Sickle Cell Disease, *Ann. Int. Med.*, **64**: 1028.
18. BLAUSTEIN, A. (1963). *The Spleen*, McGraw Hill, New York.

19. BREW, D. S. and EDINGTON, G. M. (1965). Haemoglobins S and C in Post Mortem Material in Ibadan, Nigeria. *Abnormal Haemoglobins in Africa* (Jonxis) Blackwell, Oxford.

20. BREWER, G. J., TARLOV, A. R. and ALVING, A. S. (1960). Methaemoglobin Reduction Test, A New Simple *In Vitro* Test for Identifying Primaquine-Sensitivity, *Bull. Wld. Hlth. Org.*, **22**: 633.

21. BREWER, G. J., TARLOV, A. R. and ALVING, A. S. (1962). The Methemoglobin Reduction Test for Primaquine-Type Sensitivity of Erythrocytes, *J. Am. Med. Ass.*, **180**: 386.

22. BROWNE, R. A. (1965). Anaesthesia in Patients with Sickle Cell Anaemia, *Brit. J. Anaesth.*, **37**: 181.

23. CARAYON, A., PERQUIS, P., PLASSART, H., COURBIL, H. and OUDART, J. L. (1966). Treize Cas de Falciformation avec Lésions Osseouses, Pouvoir Destructif des Divers Germes, *Bull. Soc. Med. Afr. Noire Lang. Franc.*, **11**: 93.

24. CARSON, P. E. and FRISCHER, H. (1966). Glucose-6-Phosphate Dehydrogenase Deficiency and Related Disorders of the Pentose Phosphate Pathway, *Am. J. Med.*, **41**: 744.

25. CHARACHE, S. and PAGE, D. L. (1967). Infarction of Bone Marrow in the Sickle Cell Disorders, *Ann. Int. Med.*, **67**: 1195.

26. CHARACHE, S. and RICHARDSON, S. N. (1964). Prolonged Survival of a Patient with Sickle Cell Anemia, *Arch. Int. Med.*, **113**: 844.

27. CHARNEY, E. and MILLER, G. (1964). Reticulocytopenia in Sickle Cell Disease, *Am. J. Dis. Child.*, **107**: 450.

28. CHERNOFF, A. I., SHAPLEIGH, J. B. and MOORE, C. V. (1954). Therapy of Chronic Ulceration of the Legs Associated with Sickle Cell Anemia, *J. Am. Med. Ass.*, **155**: 1487.

29. CHOREMIS, L., KATTAMIS, C. A., KYRIAZAKOU, M. and GAVRILIDOU, E. (1966). Viral Hepatitis in Glucose-6-Phosphate Dehydrogenase Deficiency, *Lancet*, **1**: 269.

30. CILIBERTI, B. J., MAZZIA, V. D. B., MARK, L. C. and MARX, G. F. (1962). Clinical Anesthesia Conference: Sickle Cell Disease and Anesthesia, *New York State J. Med.*, **62**: 548.

31. COCHRAN, R. T. Jr. (1963). Hyposthenuria in Sickle Cell States, *Arch. Int. Med.*, **112**: 222.

32. COCKSHOTT, W. P. (1965). Some Radiological Aspects of the S Haemoglobinopathies as Seen in Ibadan. *Abnormal Haemoglobins in Africa* (Jonxis) Blackwell, Oxford.

33. CURTIS, E. M. (1959). Pregnancy in Sickle Cell Anemia, Sickle Cell Hemoglobin C Disease and Variants Thereof, *Am. J. Obstet. Gynec.*, **77**: 1312.

34. DACIE, J. V. and LEWIS, S. M. (1963). *Practical Haematology*, 3rd Ed. Churchill, London.

35. DALAND, G. A. and CASTLE, W. B. (1948). A Simple and Rapid Method for, Demonstrating Sickling of Red Blood Cells: The Use of Reducing Agents, *J. Lab. Clin. Med.*, **33**: 1082.

36. DAVIS, L. J. and BROWN, A. (1953). *The Megaloblastic Anaemias*, Blackwell, Oxford.

37. DIGGS, L. W. (1965). Sickle Cell Crises, *Am. J. Clin. Path.*, **44**: 1.

38. DONEGAN, C. C., MacILWAINE, W. A. and LEAVELL, B. S. (1954). Hematologic Studies on Patients with Sickle Cell Anemia Following Multiple Transfusions, *Am. J. Med.*, **17**: 29.

39. DUNN, J. M. and HAYNES, R. L. (1967). Sickle Cell Thalassemia in Pregnancy, *Am. J. Obstet. Gynec.*, **97**: 574.

40. EGDAHL, R. H., MARTIN, W. W. and HILKOVITZ, G. (1963). Splenectomy for Hypersplenism in Sickle Cell Anemia, *J. Am. Med. Ass.*, **186**: 745.
41. EMMEL, V. E. (1917). Study of Erythrocytes in a Case of Severe Anemia with Elongated and Sickle Shaped Red Blood Corpuscles, *Arch. Int. Med.*, **20**: 586.
42. FERTMAN, M. H. and FERTMAN, M. B. (1955). Toxic Anemias and Heinz Bodies, *Medicine*, **34**: 131.
43. FULLERTON, W. T., HENDRICKSE, J. P. DeV. and WATSON-WILLIAMS, E. J. (1965). Haemoglobin SC Disease in Pregnancy—A Review of 190 Cases, *Abnormal Haemoglobins in Africa* (Jonxis) Blackwell, Oxford.
44. GALL, J. C. Jr., BREWER, G. J. and DERN, R. J. (1965). Studies of Glucose-6-Phosphate Dehydrogenase Activity of Individual Erythrocytes: The Methemoglobin Elution Test for Identification of Females Heterozygous for G6PD Deficiency, *Am. J. Human Genet.*, **17**: 359.
45. GILBERT, C. and JILLY, P. (1964). Further Observations on Factors Associated with Neonatal Jaundice in Accra, *Ghana Med. J.*, **3**: 112.
46. GILBERTSON, A. A. (1965). Anaesthesia in West African Patients with Sickle Cell Anaemia, Haemoglobin SC Disease and Sickle Cell Trait, *Brit. J. Anaesth.*, **37**: 614.
47. GILLES, H. M. and TAYLOR, B. G. (1961). The Existence of Glucose-6-Phosphate Dehydrogenase Deficiency Trait in Nigeria and its Clinical Implications, *Ann. Trop. Med. Parasitol.*, **55**: 64.
48. GOLDING, J. S. R. (1956). The Bone Changes in Sickle Cell Anaemia, *Ann. Roy. Coll. Surg.*, **19**: 296.
49. GOLDSTEIN, M. A., PATPONGPANI, J. N. and MINNICH, V. (1964). The Incidence of Elevated Hemoglobin A_2 Levels in the American Negro, *Ann. Int. Med.*, **60**: 95.
50. GRIGGS, R. C. and HARRIS, J. W. (1956). Biophysics of the Variants of Sickle Cell Disease, *Arch. Int. Med.*, **97**: 315.
51. GUERI. (1969). Cutaneous Ulcers in Sickle Cell Anaemia in Jamaica. *Blood*, **34**: 391.
52. HANSEN-PRUSS, O. C. (1936). Experimental Studies of Sickling of Red Blood Cells, *J. Lab. Clin. Med.*, **22**: 311.
53. HARRIS, J. W. (1963). *The Red Cell-Production, Metabolism, Destruction: Normal and Abnormal*, Harvard Univ. Press, Cambridge, Mass.
54. HARROW, B. R., SLOANE, J. A. and LIEBMAN, N. C. (1963). Roentgenological Demonstration of Renal Papillary Necrosis in Sickle Cell Trait, *New Eng. J. Med.*, **268**: 969.
55. HATHORN, M. (1967). Patterns of Red Cell Destruction in Sickle Cell Anaemia, *Brit. J. Haematol.*, **13**: 746.
56. HELLER, P., YAKULIS, V. J., EPSTEIN, R. B. and FRIEDLAND, S. (1963). Variation in the Amount of Hemoglobin S in a Patient with Sickle Cell Trait and Megaloblastic Anemia, *Blood*, **21**: 479.
57. HENDRICKSE, R. G. (1965). The Effect of Malaria Chemoprophylaxis on Spleen Size in Sickle Cell Anaemia, *Abnormal Haemoglobins in Africa* (Jonxis) Blackwell, Oxford.
58. HENDRICKSE, R. G. and BARNES, P. M. (1966). Sickle Cell Anaemia (Report of a Therapeutic Trial), *West African Med. J.*, **15**: 55.
59. HERRICK, J. B. (1910). Peculiar Elongated and Sickle Shaped Red Blood Corpuscles in a Case of Severe Anemia, *Arch. Int. Med.*, **6**: 517.
60. HILKOVITZ, G. and JACOBSON, A. (1961). Hepatic Dysfunction and Abnormalities of the Serum Proteins and Serum Enzymes in Sickle Cell Anemia, *J. Lab. Clin. Med.*, **57**: 856.
61. HO, PING, KONG. (1969). Acid Base Studies in Sickle Cell Anemia. *Blood*, **34**: 391.

62. HUTCHISON, H. E. (1967). *An Introduction to the Haemoglobinopathies and the Methods Used for their Recognition*, Arnold, London.

63. INGRAM, V. M. (1961). *Hemoglobin and its Abnormalities*, Thomas, Springfield, Illinois.

64. INGRAM, V. M. (1963). *The Hemoglobins in Genetics and Evolution*. Columbia Univ. Press, New York.

65. JACKSON, J. F., ODOM, J. L. and BELL, W. N. (1961). Amelioration of Sickle Cell Disease by Persistent Fetal Hemoglobin, *J. Am. Med. Ass.*, **177**: 867.

66. JANDL, J. H. and ASTER, R. H. (1967). Increased Splenic Pooling and the Pathogenesis of Hypersplenism, *Am. J. Med. Dis.*, **253**: 383.

67. JENKINS, M. E., SCOTT, R. B. and BAIRD, R. L. (1960). Studies in Sickle Cell Anemia XVI, Sudden Death During Sickle Cell Anemia Crises in Young Children, *J. Pediat.*, **56**: 30.

68. JENKINS, T. (1963). Surgical Aspects of Sickle Cell Anaemia, *Med. Proc. (South Africa)*, **9**: 6.

69. JENSEN, W. N. (1969). Electron Microscopic Studies of Sickling. *Blood.* **34**: 391.

70. JILLY, P. and NKRUMAH, F. K. (1964). A Survey of Anaemia in Children in the Korle Bu Hospital, with Special Reference to Malaria, *Ghana Med. J.*, **3**: 118.

71. JIMENEZ, C. T., SCOTT, R. B., HENRY, W. L., SAMPSON, C. C. and FERGUSON, A. D. (1966). Studies in Sickle Cell Anemia XXVI, The Effects of Homozygous Sickle Cell Disease on the Onset of Menarche, Pregnancy, Fertility, Pubescent Changes, and Body Growth in Negro Subjects, *Am. J. Dis. Child.*, **111**: 497.

72. JONXIS, J. H. P. and HUISMAN, T. H. J. (1968). *A Laboratory Manual on Abnormal Haemoglobins*, 2nd Ed. Blackwell, Oxford.

73. JORDAN, R. A. (1957). Cholelithiasis in Sickle Cell Disease, *Gastroenterol.*, **33**: 952.

74. KARBAAT, J. (1963). Het Belang van Onderzoek op Abnormale Haemoglobinen en Gebrek aan Glucose-6-Phosphaat Dehydrogenase bij de Militaire Keuring van Uit de Tropen Afkomstige Mensen, *Ned. Militair, Geneesk. Tidj.*, **16**: 200.

75. KAUFMAN, M., STEIER, W., APPLEWHAITE, F., RUGGIERO, S. and GINSBERG, V. (1965). Sickle Cell Trait in Blood Donors, *Am. J. Med. Sci.*, **249**: 56.

76. KELLERMEYER, R. W., TARLOV, A. R., BREWER, G. J., CARSON, P. E. and ALVING, A. S. (1962). Hemolytic Effect of Therapeutic Drugs: Clinical Considerations of Primaquine Type Hemolysis, *J. Am. Med. Ass.*, **180**: 388.

77. KLION, F. M., WEINER, M. J. and SCHAFFNER, F. (1964). Cholestasis in Sickle Cell Anemia, *Am. J. Med.*, **37**: 829.

78. KONOTEY-AHULU, F. I. D. (1965). Sicklaemic Human Hygrometers, *Lancet*, **1**: 1003.

79. KONOTEY-AHULU, F. I. D. and LEWIS, R. A. (1969). "Priapism in Sickle Cell States." (In Preparation).

80. LAMBOTTE-LEGRAND, J. and LAMBOTTE-LEGRAND, C. (1955). Le Prognostic de l'Anémie Drépanocytaire au Congo Belge, *Ann. Soc. Belge Méd Trop.*, **35**: 53.

81. LEHMANN, H. and HUNTSMAN, R. G. (1966). *Man's Haemoglobins*, North-Holland, Amsterdam.

82. LEVERE, R. D., LICHTMAN, H. C. and LEVINE, J. (1964). Effect of Iron Deficiency Anemia on the Metabolism of the Heterogenic Haemoglobins in Sickle Cell Trait, *Nature*, **202**: 499.

83. LEWIS, R. A. (1963). *Tropical Therapeutics: Its Pharmacologic Aspects*, Thomas, Springfield, Illinois.

84. LEWIS, R. A. (1968). Experience with Promazine in Sickle Cell Disease, *West African Med. J.*, **17**: 142.

85. LEWIS, R. A. (1967). Sickle Cell Anaemia in G-6-P D Deficiency, *Lancet*, **1**: 852.

86. LEWIS, R. A. (1967). Haematuria due to Sickling Treated with Promazine, *Brit. J. Clin. Pract.*, **21**: 139.

87. LEWIS, R. A., KAY, R. W. and HATHORN, M. (1966). Sickle Cell Disease and Glucose-6-Phosphate Dehydrogenase, *Acta Haematol*, **35**: 399.

88. LEWIS, R. A. and HAWE, A. J. (1967). Pulmonary Infarction following Air Flight in an Individual with Sickle Cell Trait, *Ghana Med. J.*, **6**: 154.

89. LEWIS, R. A. and LAHIRI, H. S. (1965). Sickle Cell Thalassaemia Treated with Promazine and Splenectomy, *Ghana Med. J.* **4**: 29.

89A. LEWIS, R. A. and LARBI, S. (1969). "Oxygen Desaturation of Incubated Blood", *Blood*, **34**: 391.

90. LIEB, W. A., GEERAETS, W. J. and GUERRY, D. III. (1959). Sickle Cell Retinopathy, Ocular and Systemic Manifestations of Sickle Cell Anemia, *Acta Ophth. Suppl.*, **58**: 7.

91. LINDENBAUM, J. and KLIPSTEIN, F. A. (1963). Folic Acid Deficiency in Sickle Cell Anemia, *New Eng. J. Med.*, **269**: 875.

92. LIVINGSTONE, F. B. (1967). *Abnormal Hemoglobins in Human Populations*, Aldine Pub. Co., Chicago.

93. LOUDERBACK, A. L. and SHANBROM, E. (1967). Hemoglobin Electrophoresis, *J. Am. Med. Ass.*, **202**: 718.

94. MACIVER, J. E., WENT, L. N. and IRVINE, R. A. (1961). Hereditary Persistence of Foetal Haemoglobin: A Family Study Suggesting Allelism of the F Genes to the S and C Haemoglobin Genes, *Brit. J. Haematol.*, **7**: 373.

95. MAFART, Y., THOMAS, J. SAGNET, M. and REVIL, H. (1966). Revue des Donées Classiques et Données Actuelles Concernant la Drépanocytose, *Méd. Trop.* **26**: 191.

96. MAHMOOD, A. (1967). The Slide Test for Sickling: A Comparison of Techniques, *Trans. Roy. Soc. Trop. Med. Hyg.*, **61**: 736.

97. MARGOLIES, M. P. (1951). Sickle Cell Anemia: A Composite Study and Survey, *Medicine*, **30**: 357.

98. MARKS, P. A. (1967). Glucose-6-Phosphate Dehydrogenase in Mature Erythrocytes, *Am. J. Clin. Path.*, **47**: 287.

99. MARSDEN, P. D. and SHAH, K. K. (1964) Artificially Induced Oedema in Sickle Cell Anaemia, *J. Trop. Med. Hyg.*, **67**: 31.

100. MARTIN, D. C. and ARNOLD, J. D. (1968). Treatment of Acute Falciparum Malaria with Sulfalene and Trimethoprim, *J. Am. Med. Ass.*, **203**: 476.

101. MONEKOSSO, G. L. and IBIAMA, A. A. (1966). Splenomegaly and Sickle Cell Trait in a Malaria Endemic Village, *Lancet*, **1**: 1347.

102. MOTULSKY, A. G. (1965). Theoretical and Clinical Problems of Glucose-6-Phosphate Dehydrogenase Deficiency: Its Occurrence in Africans and its Combination with Haemoglobinopathy. *Abnormal Haemoglobins in Africa (Jonxis)*, Blackwell, Oxford.

103. MOURANT, A. E. (1954). *Distribution of Human Blood Groups*. Blackwell, Oxford.

104. MUNRO, S. and WALKER, C. (1960). Ocular Complications in Sickle Cell Haemoglobin C Disease, *Brit. J. Ophth.*, **44**: 1.

105. MURAYAMA, M. (1966). Molecular Mechanisms of Red Cell Sickling, *Science*, **153**: 145.

106. NEEL, J. V., WELLS, I. C. and ITANO, H. A. (1951). Familial Differences in the Proportion of Abnormal Hemoglobin Present in the Sickle-Cell Trait, *J. Clin. Invest.*, **30**: 1120.

107. NG, M. L., LIEBMAN, J., ANSLOVAR, J. and GROSS, S. (1967). Cardiovascular Findings in Children with Sickle Cell Anemia, *Dis. Chest*, **52**: 788.

108. NOLL, J. B., NEWMAN, A. J. and GROSS, S. (1967). Enuresis and Nocturia in Sickle Cell Disease, *J. Pediat.*, **70**: 965.

109. O'FLYNN, M. E. D. and HSIA, Y. Y. D. (1963). Serum Bilirubin Levels and Glucose-6-Phosphate Dehydrogenase Deficiency in New Born American Negroes, *J.Pediat.*, **63**: 160.

110. OSKI, F., CALL, F. L. II and LESSEN, L. (1968). Failure of Promazine HCl to Prevent the Painful Episodes in Sickle Cell Anemia, *J. Pediat.*, **73**: 265.

111. OSKI, F. A., VINER, E. D., PURUGGANAN, H. and MCELFRESH, A. E. (1965). Low Molecular Weight Dextran in Sickle Cell Crisis, *J. Am. Med. Ass.*, **191**: 43.

112. OWEN, D. M., ALDRIDGE, J. E. and THOMPSON, R. B. (1965). An Unusual Hepatic Sequela of Sickle Cell Anemia, A Report of 5 Cases, *Am. J. Med. Sci.*, **249**: 175.

113. PATERSON, J. C. S. and SPRAGUE, C. C. (1959). Observations on the Genesis of Crises in Sickle Cell Anemia, *Ann. Int. Med.*, **50**: 1502.

114. PATTERSON, R. J., BICKEL, W. H. and DAHLIN, D. C. (1964). Idiopathic Avascular Necrosis of the Head of the Femur, *J. Bone Joint Surg.*, **46A**: 267.

115. PAULING, L. (1955). Abnormality of Hemoglobin Molecules in Hereditary Hemolytic Anemia, *Harvey Lecture Series*, **49**: 216.

116. PEARSON, H. A. and COBB, W. T. (1964). Folic Acid Studies in Sickle-Cell Anemia, *J. Lab. Clin. Med.*, **64**: 913.

117. PERUTZ, M. F. (1962). *Proteins and Nucleic Acids—Structure and Function*. Elsevier Pub. Co., Amsterdam.

118. PIETERS, G. et LAMBOTTE, C. (1965). La Pathologie Chirurgicale de la Sicklanémie, *Abnormal Haemoglobins in Africa (Jonxis)*, Blackwell, Oxford.

119. PINKERTON, P. H. and COHEN, M. M. (1967). Persistence of Hemoglobin F in D/D Translocation with Trisomy 13–15 (D₁), *J. Am. Med. Ass.*, **200**: 647.

120. PORTER, F. S. and THURMAN, W. G. (1963). Studies of Sickle Cell Disease, *Am. J. Dis. Child.*, **106**: 35.

121. RAPER, A. B. (1956). Sickling in Relation to Morbidity from Malaria and Other Diseases, *Brit. Med. J.*, **1**: 965.

122. RAPER, A. B. (1968). A Commentary on the Anti-Sickling Effect of the Phenothiazine Drugs, *Trans. Roy. Soc. Trop. Med. Hyg.*, **62**: 84.

123. RAPER, A. B. (1969). The "Simple" Slide Test for Sickling, *Ghana Med. J.*, **8**: 29.

124. RATCLIFF, R. G. and WOLF, M. D. (1962). Avascular Necrosis of the Femoral Head Associated with Sickle Cell Trait, *Ann. Int. Med.*, **57**: 299.

125. Report of a WHO Drafting Committee. (1963). Terminology of Malaria and Malaria Eradication, *Wld. Hlth. Org.*, Geneva.

126. Report of a WHO Scientific Group. (1966). "Haemoglobinopathies and Allied Disorders." WHO Technical Report Series No. 338, Geneva.

127. Report of a WHO Scientific Group. (1967). "Standardization of Procedures for the Study of Glucose-6-Phosphate Dehydrogenase." WHO Technical Report Series No. 366, Geneva.

128. REYNOLDS, J. (1965). *The Roentgenological Features of Sickle Cell Disease and Related Hemoglobinopathies*, Thomas, Springfield, Illinois.

129. RINGELHANN, B., DODU, S. R. A., KONOTEY-AHULU, F. I. D. and LEHMANN, H. (1968). A Survey for Haemoglobin Variants, Thalassaemia and Glucose-6-Phosphate Dehydrogenase Deficiency in Northern Ghana, *Ghana Med. J.* **7**: 120.

130. RINGELHANN, B., LEWIS, R. A., LORKIN, D. A., KYNOCH, P. A. M. and LEHMANN, H. (1967). Sickle Cell Haemoglobin D Punjab Disease: S from Ghana and D from England, *Acta Haematologica*, **38**: 324.

131. ROBIN, H. and HARLEY, J. D. (1966). Experience with an Extended Methemoglobin Reduction Test, *Blood*, **27**: 395.

132. ROBINSON, M. G. and WATSON, R. J. (1966). Pneumococcal Meningitis in Sickle Cell Anemia, *New Eng. J. Med.*, **274**: 1006.

133. ROSENBAUM, J. M. (1965). Fatal Hemoglobin S-C Disease Crisis Following Tonsillectomy, *Arch. Otolaryng.*, **82**: 307.

134. ROTTER, R., LUTGENS, W. F., PETERSON, W. L., STOCK, A. E. and MOTULSKY, A. G. (1956). Splenic Infarction in Sicklemia during Airplane Flight, *Ann. Int. Med.*, **44**: 257.

135. RUCKNAGEL, D. L. and NEEL, J. V. (1961). The Hemoglobinopathies, *Progress in Medical Genetics*, **1**: 158.

136. RUSSELL, P. F., WEST, L. S., MANWELL, R. D. and MacDONALD, G. (1963). *Practical Malariology*, 2nd Ed. Oxford, London.

137. RYWLIN, A. M., BLOCK, A. L. and WERNER, C. S. (1963). Hemoglobin C and S Disease in Pregnancy, Report of a Case with Bone Marrow and Fat Emboli, *Am. J. Obstet. Gynec.*, **86**: 1055.

138. SAGNET, A., LEVOURCH, C., DELPRAT, J., REVIL, H., THOMAS, J. and MARFAT, Y. (1969). Les Thalasso-Drépanocytoses, *Med. Trop.*, **28**: 591.

139. SALEN, G., GOLDSTEIN, F., HAURANI, F. and WIRTS, C. W. (1966). Acute Hemolytic Anemia Complicating Viral Hepatitis in Patients with Glucose-6-Phosphate Dehydrogenase Deficiency, *Ann. Int. Med.*, **65**: 1210.

140. SALVAGGIO, J. E., ARNOLD, C. A. and BANOV, C. H. (1963). Long Term Anticoagulant Therapy in Sickle Cell Disease: Clinical Study, *New Eng. J. Med.*, **269**: 182.

141. SALVIDIO, E., PANNACCIULLI, I. and TIZIANELLO, A. (1963). Glucose-6-Phosphate Dehydrogenase Deficiency in Sardinians, *Proc. IX Cong. Europ. Soc. Haematol.*, Lisbon.

142. SCHNEIDER, R. G., ALPERIN, J. B. and LEHMANN, H. (1967). Sickling Tests, Pitfalls in Performance and Interpretation, *J. Am. Med. Ass.*, **202**: 117.

143. SCHWARTZ, E. and McELFRESH, A. C. (1964). Treatment of Painful Crisis of Sickle Cell Disease, A Double Blind Study, *J. Pediat.*, **64**: 132.

144. SERJEANT, G. (1969). "Sickle Cell Anemia in Jamaica." *Blood*, **34**: 391.

145. SHERMAN, I. J. (1940). The Sickling Phenomenon with Special Reference to the Differentiation of Sickle Cell Anemia from Sickle Cell Trait, *Bull. Johns Hopkins Hosp.*, **67**: 309.

146. SHERMAN, M. (1959). Pathogenesis of Disintegration of the Hip in Sickle Cell Anemia, *South. Med. J.*, **52**: 632.

147. SINGER, K., ROBINS, S., KING, J. C. and JEFFERSON, R. N. (1949). The Life Span of the Sickle Cell and the Pathogenesis of Sickle Cell Anemia, *J. Lab. Clin. Med.*, **33**: 975.

148. SMITH, C. H. (1966). *Blood Diseases of Infancy and Childhood*, 2nd Ed Mosby, St. Louis.

149. SMITH, C. H., ERLANDSON, M. E., SCHULMAN, I. and STERN, G. (1957). Hazard of Severe Infection in Splenectomized Infants, *Am. J. Med.*, **22**: 390.

150. SMITH, E. W. and CONLEY, C. L. (1954). Clinical Features of the Genetic Variants of Sickle Cell Disease, *Bull. Johns Hopkins Hosp.*, **94**: 289.

151. SMITH, E. W. and CONLEY, C. L. (1955). Sicklemia and Infarction of the Spleen during Aerial Flight, *Bull. Johns Hopkins Hosp.*, **96**: 35.

152. SMITH, I. (1960). *Chromatographic and Electrophoretic Techniques*, Vol. II, Zone Electrophoresis, Interscience Pub. Corp., New York.

153. SPECIAL CORRESPONDENT. (1967). Tropical Splenomegaly Syndrome, *Brit. Med. J.*, **4**: 614.

154. SPRAGUE, C. C. and PATERSON, J. C. S. (1958). The Role of the Spleen and Effect of Splenectomy in Sickle Cell Disease, *Blood*, **13**: 569.

155. STONE, H. H., STANLEY, D. G. and DEFARNETTE, R. H. (1967). Postsplenectomy Viral Hepatitis, *J. Am. Med. Ass.*, **199**: 851.

156. SUNDERMAN, F. W. and SUNDERMAN, F. W. Jr. (1964). *Hemoglobin: Its Precursors and Metabolites*, Lippincott, Philadelphia.

157. TARLOV, A. R., BREWER, G. J., CARSON, P. E. and ALVING, A. S. (1962). Primaquine Sensitivity—Glucose-6-Phosphate Dehydrogenaze Deficiency, an Inborn Error of Metabolism of Medical and Biological Significance, *Arch. Int. Med.*, **109**: 209.

158. THOMPSON, R. B. and HOLLOWAY, C. H. (1963). Observations on the Sickling Phenomenon, *Am. J. Med. Technol.*, **29**: 379.

159. TOMLINSON, W. J. (1945). Abdominal Crises in Uncomplicated Sickle Cell Anemia: A Clinicopathologic Study of 11 Cases with a Suggested Explanation of their Cause, *Am. J. Med. Sci.*, **209**: 722.

160. TROWELL, H. C., RAPER, A. B. and WELBOURN, R. F. (1957). The Natural History of Homozygous Sickle-Cell Anaemia in Central Africa, *Quart. J. Med.*, **26**: 401.

161. TRUONG, T. B., FERGUSON, A. D., BOOKER, C. R. and SCOTT, R. B. (1964). Growth and Development of Negro Infants: X, Fetal Hemoglobin in Sicklers and Non-Sicklers During the First Two Years of Life, *Am. J. Dis. Child.*, **107**: 25.

162. VARDY, P. A. and HERSHKO, C. (1967). Haemolysis in Typhoid Fever in Children with Glusose-6-Phosphate Dehydrogenase Deficiency, *Brit. Med. J.*, **1**: 214.

163. VEIGA, S. and VAITHIANATHAN, T. (1963). Massive Intravenous Sickling After Exchange Transfusion with Sickle Cell Trait Blood, *Transfusion*, **3**: 387.

164. WALTERS, J. (1964). The Surgical Aspects of Sickle Cell Anaemia, *Proc. Roy. Soc. Med.*, **57**: 1147.

165. WARLEY, M. A., HAMILTON, P. J. S., MARSDEN, P. D., BROWN, R. E., MERSELIS, J. E. and WILKS, N. (1965). Chemoprophylaxis of Homozygous Sicklers with Antimalarials and Long Acting Penicillin, *Brit. Med. J.*, **2**: 86.

166. WATSON, R. J., BURKO, H., MEGAS, H. and ROBINSON, M. (1963). The Hand Foot Syndrome in Sickle Cell Disease in Young Children, *Pediatrics*, **31**: 975.

167. WATSON-WILLIAMS, E. J. (1965). The Role of Folic Acid in the Treatment of Sickle Cell Disease, *Abnormal Haemoglobins in Africa* (Jonxis), Blackwell, Oxford.

168. WEATHERALL, D. J. (1968). *The Thalassaemia Syndromes*, 2nd Ed. Blackwell, Oxford.

169. WESSLER, S. and AVIOLI, L. V. (1968). Pharmacogenetics, *J. Am. Med. Ass.*, **205**: 679.

170. WHALLEY, P. J., MARTIN, F. G. and PRITCHARD, J. A. (1964). Sickle Cell Trait and Urinary Tract Infection During Pregnancy, *J. Am. Med. Ass.*, **189**: 903.

171. WINTROBE, M. M. (1961). *Clinical Hematology*, 5th Ed. Klimpton, London.

172. WORLD HEALTH ORGANIZATION. (1961). Chemotherapy of Malaria, Tech. Report Series No. **226**.

173. WORLD HEALTH ORGANIZATION. (1959). Iron Deficiency Anaemia, Tech. Report Series No. **182**.

174. ZINKHAM, W. H. and CHILDS, R. (1958). Metabolism in Erythrocytes from Patients with a Naphthalene-Induced Hemolytic Anemia, *Pediatrics*, **22**: 461.

Index